Teamwork in Neurology

THERAPY IN PRACTICE SERIES
Edited by Jo Campling

This series of books is aimed at 'therapists' concerned with rehabilitation in a very broad sense. The intended audience particularly includes occupational therapists, physiotherapists and speech and language therapists, but many titles will also be of interest to nurses, psychologists, medical staff, social workers, teachers or volunteer workers. Some volumes are interdisciplinary, others are aimed at one particular profession. All titles will be comprehensive but concise, and practical but with due reference to relevant theory and evidence. They are not research monographs but focus on professional practice, and will be of value to both students and qualified personnel.

A manual for writers
Philip Burnard
33. Brain Injury Rehabilitation
A neuro-functional approach
Gordon Muir Giles and Jo Clark-Wilson
34. Living with Continuing Percepto-motor Difficulties
Theory and strategies to help children, adolescents and adults
Dorothy E. Penso
35. Psychology and Counselling for Health Professionals
Edited by Rowan Bayne and Paula Nicholson
36. Occupational Therapy for Orthopaedic Conditions
Dina Penrose
37. Teaching Students in Clinical Settings
Jackie Stengelhofen
38. Group work in Occupational Therapy
Linda Finlay
39. Elder Abuse
Concepts, theories and interventions
Gerald Bennett and Paul Kingston
40. Teamwork in Neurology
Ruth Nieuwenhuis
41. Eating Disorders
A guide for professionals
Simon Thompson
42. Community Mental Health
Practical approaches to the long-term problems
Steve Morgan

FORTHCOMING TITLES
Research Methods for Therapists
Avril Drummond

Stroke: Recovery and Rehabilitation
Polly Laidler

HIV and Aids Care
S. Singh and L. Cusack

Speech and Language Disorders in Children
Dilys A. Treharne

Spinal Cord Rehabilitation
Karen Whalley-Hammell

Teamwork in Neurology

Ruth Nieuwenhuis
MA(Hons), Dip CSLT, Reg MCSLT
Sully Hospital Stroke Unit, South Glamorgan

CHAPMAN & HALL
London · Glasgow · New York · Tokyo · Melbourne · Madras

Published by Chapman & Hall, 2–6 Boundary Row, London SE1 8HN

Chapman & Hall, 2–6 Boundary Row, London SE1 8HN, UK

Blackie Academic & Professional, Wester Cleddens Road, Bishopbrigg, Glasgow G6 2NZ, UK

Chapman & Hall Inc., 29 West 35th Street, New York NY10001, USA

Chapman & Hall Japan, Thomson Publishing Japan, Hirakawacho Building, 6F, 1–7–11 Hirakawa-cho, Chiyoda-ku, Tokyo 102 Japan

Chapman & Hall Australia, Thomas Nelson Australia, 102 Dodds Street, South Melbourne, Victoria 3205, Australia

Chapman & Hall India, R. Seshadri, 32 Second Main Road, CIT East, Madras 600 035, India

Distributed in the USA and Canada by Singular Publishing Group Inc., 4284 41st Street, San Diego, California 92105

First edition 1993

© 1993 Ruth Nieuwenhuis
Phototypeset in 10/12pt Palatino by Intype, London

Printed in Great Britain by Page Bros, Norwich

ISBN 0 412 39350 6 ✓   1 56593 121 1 (USA)

A catalogue record for this book is available from the British Library

Library of Congress Cataloging-in-Publication data available.

∞ Printed on permanent acid-free text paper, manufactured in accordance with the proposed ANSI/NISO Z 39.48–199X and ANSI Z 39.48–1984

Contents

Preface

The problems which hamper teamwork in health care are well-documented. Foremost among these is a lack of knowledge about each others' professions linked with poor understanding and misperception of each others' roles. Limited appreciation of the vital contributions of both patient and family is another important factor.

This book aims to address these and other issues, thereby encouraging improvements in the quality of health care. It developed from an interest in teamwork with adults who had suffered brain damage due to trauma, neurological illness or degenerative neurological disease. The text reflects many years of practical experience gained both in hospitals and in the community. It assumes that shared knowledge between the professions may promote greater mutual understanding and foster positive working relations.

Some stylistic features require explanation. The use of 'he' and 'she' is always problematical. Ideally, both pronouns should be used simultaneously because there are male or female individuals in all walks of life. However the repeated use of 'he/she' becomes unwieldy and I have adopted, therefore, the following convention: 'he' refers to patients and doctors and 'she' to nurses, physiotherapists, occupational therapists, speech and language therapists, dieticians, social workers and clinical psychologists.

Another important point concerns different terminology in the UK and the US. A 'physiotherapist' in Britain is known as a 'physical therapist' in the States. Similarly, a 'speech and language therapist' is known as a 'speech and language pathologist'. Some of these different terms appear in the book, their use dictated by the context. Furthermore, all patients' names have been changed.

I would like to thank my colleagues who shared their practical expertise and provided help and support. Particular thanks go to those at the James Paget Hospital, Gorleston, Great Yarmouth – namely Elizabeth Burningham, occupational therapist, and Linda Clarke, physiotherapist. Staff at the 'Stroke Unit' at the University Hospital of Wales have also been very helpful, especially Maggie Gillingham, dietician; Jennifer Moses, clinical psychologist; Margaret Moss, social worker; Delyth Rees, occupational therapist; and Maggie Webster, physiotherapist. Barbara McCaffer and Helen Hughes, dieticians at Sully Hospital, near Cardiff gave very useful information, whilst Andrew Butcher (formerly Unit General Manager at the James Paget Hospital) arranged financial support for the necessary library research. Christine Thompson, librarian there, carried this out along with Alan Bullimore. Both willingly shared their knowledge and expertise.

Finally, Paul and Mum and Dad sustained the project from start to finish. This book is dedicated to all three.

Ruth Nieuwenhuis

1

Introduction

We each secretly believe that our profession has the most to offer.

Fussey and Giles, 1988, p. 184.

THE LITERATURE ON TEAMWORK

For years, teamwork has been a popular subject in health care. A wealth of literature exists extolling the benefits gained by both patients and staff when professionals manage to work together. Articles and books abound. Words such as 'interdisciplinary', 'transdisciplinary', 'multidisciplinary', and 'team building' recur regularly on both sides of the Atlantic. There is even debate about the definitions of these terms. A common theme is the need for those who work in health care to understand each others' roles. This allows individuals with different jobs to work effectively together as a unified body.

The current literature on the topic (with regard to the adult with acquired neurological brain damage) consists of both general and specific professional texts as well as scores of articles. The general texts are aimed at all members of the rehabilitation team, often containing contributions from members of individual professions. Some deal with neurological rehabilitation as a whole, others with particular neurological conditions, such as head injury.

A good example of this type of book is Fussey and Giles (1988). It provides excellent coverage of rehabilitation of the severely brain-injured adult. The authors advocate a behavioural treatment approach to the post-acute patient. Another example is Garner (1990) who covers rehabilitation of acute head injury. Other works include: Cochrane (1987), who focuses on the management of motor neurone disease; Caird

(1991), who looks at rehabilitation in Parkinson's Disease; Maloney *et al.* (1985) who cover multiple sclerosis and neuromuscular disorders.

Several texts are devoted purely to stroke rehabilitation (Wade *et al.*, 1985; Branstater and Basmajian, 1987; Allen *et al.*, 1988). Some of these, despite their claims, are poor advertisements for teamwork. The contributors in Kaplan and Cerullo (1986), for example, frequently cover the same area of practice without sufficient reference to each other. The nurses in Chapter 12 and the physical therapists in Chapter 14 both discuss bed positioning. They are obviously experts in their own fields but they acknowledge neither the involvement nor the expertise of each other. This suggests that they work completely separately. Inevitably the casualty is the patient. Johnstone (1987) is another text devoted to teamwork within stroke rehabilitation. Unfortunately she adopts a heavy physiotherapy bias, despite her title *The Stroke Patient: A Team Approach*. She also fails to support her remarks with proven references.

Texts written by doctors also advocate teamwork. Understandably, however, they have little to say about how to achieve this in practical therapy sessions. Their remarks reflect their medical training and expertise. They write from the doctor's point of view (Ashworth and Saunders, 1985) and some have rather set views on the work of the paramedical and nursing professions (Wade *et al.*, 1985; Allen *et al.*, 1988).

The other section of the literature – specific professional texts – tends to be written by and for individuals in a particular discipline. Their very titles contain terms such as 'nursing' (Dittmar, 1989) and 'occupational therapy' (Eggers, 1988; Hopkins and Smith, 1988). Hence people outside those professions may be unfamiliar with them. This means that the valuable information they contain on teamwork remains inaccessible to other professionals. This is unfortunate because these individuals are the very people who will make up the team, influencing its success.

And what about the patient and his family? Most recent texts on teamwork agree that their involvement is crucial for the success of treatment. Yet, with a few exceptions, many say little about identifying their needs or about the practicalities of working together to meet these. Indeed the patient is often the last on the list of possible team members. Despite this, patients and members of their families are the people most qualified to talk about the problems they experience. Many have put pen to paper and tried to convey how they feel. They have written articles and letters about their difficulties, sometimes complaining about the services they receive (see Chapter 2).

Unfortunately, they do not have access to learned medical journals and professional texts. Their anecdotal accounts fail to qualify as essential reading for the busy doctor, nurse and paramedic. Thus their words appear in lay publications, consulted by the staff who treat them, only as an afterthought, if at all. For this and other reasons, self-help groups have evolved both in the UK and the US. There are individual societies devoted to stroke, head injury, Alzheimer's disease and multiple sclerosis to name just a few.

THE AIM OF THIS BOOK

This book will attempt to address some of the issues highlighted above. It will share information between members of certain professions who work with adults with acquired neurological brain damage. These will include doctors, nurses, physiotherapists, occupational therapists, speech and language therapists, dieticians, social workers, clinical psychologists as well as various types of paramedical helper or assistant. The sharing of information is designed to facilitate the understanding of each others' roles.

In addition the text will aim, at all times, to be readable and easily understood. This is an important consideration. Reading a book, or parts of it, is heavy going when there are long sentences, obscure in meaning. These frequently distance the reader from the message. Nevertheless many academics confuse a heavy and turgid writing style with academic excellence (Burnard, 1990, p. 19). Accordingly, this book will try to be as user-friendly as possible. Its content is based on a survey and analysis of the relevant literature and personal clinical experience. This has been gained over a number of years of work, both in hospitals and in the community, with the adult with acquired neuorological brain damage.

This initial chapter discusses further the concept of teamwork. In addition, it outlines some of the main causes of acquired brain damage in adults. Chapter 2 surveys a selection of the literature of various self-help groups, pinpointing several recurrent themes. These have implications for the professional at work. The next chapter looks at the historical background of certain disciplines, identifying the pressures which bear down on individual members of the team. Assessment is covered in Chapter 4. Topics include a discussion of areas of overlap and possible ways of improving communication.

Chapter 5 summarizes several approaches to health care. It also describes some of the different models and techniques which are used. Once again identification of areas of overlap leads to a discussion of the implications for both the patient and the working professional. Obviously education and training are crucial and these are the subjects of Chapter 6. Chapters 7 and 8 illustrate the 'nuts and bolts' of teamwork. They contain practical hospital and community case histories, drawn directly from personal clinical experience. Both successful outcomes and difficult problems are discussed. The final chapter offers some conclusions and recommedations.

ACHIEVING TEAMWORK

Edwards and Hanley (1989) summarize the advantages of teamwork rather well: teamwork makes service delivery more efficient; it exposes professionals to novel aims and methods of assessment and management; it unites them and enhances their potential to influence a change of policy; and it improves their professional situation. We can add to this two further benefits: teamwork can lead colleagues to develop new ideas about how to actually treat the patient (Fussey and Giles, 1988); and it can reduce the relatives' chances of misunderstanding what they have been told (Eames and Wood, 1989).

Despite the obvious advantages, actually achieving successful, cohesive teamwork may be difficult. Often, joint efforts to help the patient may resemble the fable of the blind man touching the elephant. His descriptions vary according to which part of the animal he feels. Thus the elephant may be 'a huge leaf waving in the breeze', 'a broad table top', 'a short dangling rope', 'a twisting snake', 'a wide wall', 'a tree trunk', or 'a spear' (adapted from Weiner, 1968). Just as the blind man fails to perceive the different bits of the animal as part of a whole, so professionals may fail to perceive the different disabilities of the patient as part of the whole person. Or they may interpret the same disability in different ways.

Compartmentalizing the patient occurs because, according to the biomedical model, the body is divided into various systems (see Chapters 4 and 5). To promote a more holistic approach, Baldwin and Hopcroft (1987) offer sound advice to newly qualified junior hospital doctors. They warn against dividing a patient up into parts.

> Regardless of the chosen speciality of the consultant responsible, it is negligent to regard his patients as possessing a particular 'system' (for example central nervous system, gastrointestinal system, etc.) with secondary anatomical appendages, such as a head: all patients, medical and surgical, should be examined as thoroughly as possible (p. 27)

Examples of a disjointed approach to patient care frequently occur. Consider, for example, a nurse who is concerned about her patient's comfort in bed. She may position several pillows at his back and around his head. This action may irritate the physiotherapist because it contributes to increased tone in the patient's affected arm. On top of this dispute different priorities may exist for yet other members of the team. The speech and language therapist, for example, may continue her sessions at the bedside without worrying about body tone at all. In this example each professional has a different view of what is most important for the patient: priorities range from comfort (the nurse) to reduction of muscle tone (the physiotherapist) to assessment of communicative skills (the speech and language therapist). Probably each person feels they MUST exercise their professional skill. Otherwise their specialist expertise will remain unrecognized.

Consider a further scenario. A young head-injured adolescent in a persistent vegetative state may show signs of beginning to swallow. The nurses may be the first to notice this when they carry out his regular mouth care. The patient may, for example, open his mouth further and bite on the glycerine stick they use. After drawing this to the attention of the consultant in charge (who may be a physician or general surgeon rather than a specialist in head injury), they may be given the go-ahead to try feeding the patient. Meanwhile the speech and language therapist may assess swallowing ability separately and decide that the patient is at risk of aspiration. Although he is now beginning to open his mouth, he may be unable to cough or protect his airway. Accordingly, she may recommend that he remain 'nil-by-mouth' in the interests of safety. Nurses and consultant may ignore her recommendations and start giving the patient sips of water and small amounts of puréed food.

In this case, the patient's family falls victim to a professional territorial dispute. While the different parties wage war about who is the expert, the patient's family struggles to interpret contradictory professional opinions – knowing throughout that they have the least specialist knowledge of the lot. Obviously these are extreme examples of disjointed teamwork. They highlight a breakdown in communication, recognized, no doubt, by most readers. Situations like this do occur, however, even in places which profess to follow a 'team' approach. The patient falls helplessly in between the cracks.

To improve patient care, at least in the field of stroke, Stevens (1989) argues in favour of stroke units. This involves rehabilitating stroke patients in one centre, rather than on medical and geriatric wards throughout a hospital. One advantage of this is that the patient receives the full attention of an enthusiastic team. Wade (1989) argues that stroke patients should be concentrated in one or two wards of district hospitals. Dittmar (1989) claims that to run smoothly, a team must have rules or formalized procedure manuals.

The vast majority of nurses and therapists do not, however, have access to this level of organization. While learned and distinguished doctors and health managers argue about policy, the nurse and 'grass-roots' recently qualified paramedic must simply get on with the job. The community professional is in a particularly difficult position. Her only point of contact with other members of the team may be the patient's home. Her headquarters may be in a completely different location from everyone else's. Indeed she may never even see her team colleagues at all. Thus in both the hospital and the community, there may be no established team as such. Moreover the individual may have neither the status, experience nor the resources to form one. She may simply have to try and get on with other people on an *ad hoc* basis.

BLURRING OF PROFESSIONAL ROLES

Of course, there are places where teams do work and, more recently, 'blurring of professional roles' has been in vogue (Fussey and Giles, 1988; Eames and Wood, 1989). This tries to avoid situations such as those described above. It involves sharing of treatment techniques and blending skills together (Wilson and Laidler, 1990). For it to work well, different staff need to agree on what is the most important priority for the patient at any one time. Furthermore all professions must work on these agreed priorities rather than concentrating on their own professional territory.

Senner-Hurley and Lefkowitz (1982) in the US provide an example of working in this way. They discuss a dysarthric patient who needs to be able to improve his breath support. Firstly the physical therapists and the speech-language pathologist work on deep breathing exercises. Then the occupational therapist offers her expertise by providing the appropriate splinting and bracing techniques which affect posture and positioning. These, along with the physical therapist's efforts to improve neck and trunk control, result in a better physiological support for speech – which, in turn, helps the speech-language pathologist at work.

Of course the patient, if he is able, and his relatives, need to agree with the therapists' aims if this approach is to work. There is no point in spending vast amounts of time and energy on trying to get them to do something they do not wish to. Such attempts are doomed to failure because the patient has neither the incentive nor the motivation. Morton (1990b) describes what can happen if the patient's opinion is ignored. She suffered a stroke and, several years later, recounted her experiences. This is how she felt when the aims of other well-meaning helpers were not the same as her own. 'It was rather like somebody else trying to help by drinking my medicine for me' (p. 6).

CAUSES OF ACQUIRED NEUROLOGICAL IMPAIRMENT IN ADULTS

The following sections summarize some of the main causes of acquired neurological brain damage in adults. Where possible, incidence and prevalence figures are given (see Appendix B: Glossary).

Stroke

A stroke or cerebrovascular accident (CVA) occurs when there is a serious, spontaneous disturbance of the blood supply to the brain. This does not include cases of trauma or surgical ligation of the blood vessels. A stroke may be ischaemic or haemorrhagic in origin. Risk factors associated with stroke include hypertension, cigarette smoking, high blood cholesterol, being overweight, ageing, and, for women, use of the contraceptive pill. Certain diseases also increase the risk of stroke, particularly those linked with arterial disease (e.g. heart failure, diabetes and so on.)

Approximately 100 000 first-ever strokes occur in Britain each year (two per 1000 population). One in four occur in people under 65 years old. A district with a population of 250 000 can expect to see 500 (0.2%) first-ever and 100 (0.04%) recurrent stroke cases per year (University of Leeds, 1992).

Ischaemic Stroke

An ischaemic stroke occurs when the blood supply to a part of the brain suddenly becomes inadquate and the brain cells can no longer function properly. This may be caused by a cerebral thrombosis (a clot which blocks a blood vessel in the brain) or an embolus. An embolus refers to a piece of clot, formed in a blood vessel outside the brain, which has broken off, been carried to the brain by the bloodstream and blocked a blood vessel there. If the damage is transient, lasting only a few minutes, the episode is known as a transient ischaemic attack.

Ischaemia results in cerebral infarction: the area of brain supplied by the affected blood vessel becomes short of blood; the cells within this either die or are temporarily knocked out of action. Hence the signs and symptoms of cerebral infarction are directly related to the area of affected brain and its damaged cells. There may be a sudden or rapid onset of paralysis, loss of sensation, loss of part of the field of vision, incontinence, difficulty in swallowing, impairment of speech, understanding, reading and writing, or all of these. Cognitive deficits may also occur, for example difficulties in attention and concentration. Recovery may begin after hours or even days. Most recovery occurs in the first few weeks but it continues until at least 6 months poststroke (Allen *et al.*, 1988). The first 3 months of recovery occur regardless of any rehabilitation given and it is most unusual for improvement to continue beyond 1 year after stroke (University of Leeds, 1992).

Haemorrhagic Strokes

In a haemorrhagic stroke there is a rupture of the wall of a blood vessel. In a **cerebral haemorrage** blood rushes into and through the brain, destroying tissue on its way. In the case of **intracerebral haematoma**, it forms a clot in the substance of the brain. In **subarachnoid haemorrage** (caused by cerebral aneurysms or cerebral angiomas) it rushes outside the brain into the subarachnoid space. Any combination of these types of haemorrhagic stroke may occur. Signs and symptoms of haemorrhagic stroke include sudden onset, headache, vomiting, rapid loss of consciousness (usually) and paralysis.

Much of this section is based on Bickerstaff (1978). More detailed information on stroke is available in Allen *et al.* (1988), Mulley (1985) and Wade *et al.* (1985).

Head injury

Head injuries may be closed (where, though the skull may be fractured, the coverings of the brain remain intact) or open (the brain or meninges are exposed). In a simple fissure skull fracture, there is no break in the skin. Compound fractures mean that the scalp is also breached whereas comminuted fractures are even more extensive, with the bone being broken into several pieces. In a depressed fracture, a piece of bone is driven inwards.

Garner (1990) outlines the extent of the problem referring to a report by the Medical Disability Society's working party (1987): the annual incidence of severe head injury is about 8/100 000 in the UK with two of these, 6 months after injury, still being in the stage of severe disability or coma. Moderate head injury occurs at a rate of about 18/100 000 per annum.

Wade and Langton Hewer (1987), however, note that there

is no secure information on the prevalance of patients disabled by head injury. The lack of any information on the use of hospital resources is almost as bad. They advocate further investigation on the management and outcome of head injury of all grades of severity. Head injury occurs commonly in young males between 15 and 22 years.

Most head injuries, however, are not penetrating wounds. The brain is damaged because it has been shaken about inside the skull. Rotational forces cause a shearing of its structures creating diffuse axonal damage. Several areas may be contused with damage to frontal and temporal poles and to the brainstem which houses the reticular formation. This network of cells and fibres is responsible for keeping the brain in a state of activity and the individual in a stake of wakefulness. Hence, a severe head injury with damage to the brainstem causes a transient loss of consciousness – or concussion. After the initial injury, secondary problems can develop. These include raised intracranial pressure, hypoxia/anoxia, or infection if the skull has been fractured. Surgical evacuation of extradural and subdural haematomas may be necessary.

The severity of acute head injury is measured in most specialist units by the Glasgow Coma Scale. This categorizes the levels of responsiveness following head injury. It assigns scores for eye opening, best verbal response and best motor response and adds them together. A score of 15 represents the most responsive whilst a score of three is the least responsive (Jennet et al., 1979). Duration of coma and length of post-traumatic amnesia (PTA) are other measures used to assess the severity of brain injury. Post-traumatic amnesia is defined as the time between injury and return to full consciousness. The longer the PTA, the more severe the injury.

After head injury, some patients recover completely and are able to carry on their lives as before. Others may continue to show symptoms attributable to the injury more than 2 years afterwards. These may include physical disorders such as paresis, dysphasia, poor coordination and so forth as well as cognitive deficits such as poor memory and concentration and lack of insight. There may also be behavioural problems (aggression, apathy and so forth) and social difficulties. Patients who recover consciousness may remain dependent upon care for the rest of their lives because damage to the brain has been so great. Some patients may lie in a coma for weeks, months and even years.

Further information on head injury is available in Brooks (1984), Fussey and Giles (1988) and Garner (1990).

Multiple sclerosis (MS)

Multiple sclerosis is a disease of the central nervous system. It involves inflammation of parts of the myelin sheath, a fatty substance which protects and insulates the axon of a nerve. Patches of demyelination called 'plaques' develop in part of the spinal cord, cerebellum, brainstem and cerebral hemispheres or optic pathways. This damage interferes with the ability of the axon to conduct impulses between the brain and the body via the spinal cord.

The inflammation may die down leaving no permanent damage. However if it continues the myellin sheath is destroyed at the point of attack. This leaves fibrous scar tissue known as plaques or sclerosis. The demyelination process typically affects more than one area of the central nervous system at different times – hence the term multiple sclerosis. The disease may present as a series of relapses and remissions or as a chronic progression. During a relapse, new symptoms occur or existing symptoms get worse. This is caused by the development of either new areas of demyelination, or the extension of an old one.

Relapses can last from a few days to many months and may be slight or severe. Remissions occur spontaneously although sometimes they are prompted by drug therapy, e.g. steroids. Recovery during a period of remission may be incomplete. When only partial recovery occurs after each relapse, the overall condition of the patient will gradually worsen. Those who have chronically progressive multiple sclerosis have symptoms which worsen gradually all the time.

Symptoms vary depending on which nerves are affected. They may include any of the following, either alone or in combination: blurring or complete loss of vision in one eye, paralysis of eye movement and diplopia, nystagmus, numbness, weakness, spasticity, ataxia, dysarthria, or bladder and bowel disturbances (frequency, urgency and urinary incontinence, retention of urine and constipation). Fatigue, problems with memory and concentration and depression may also occur.

The cause of the disease remains unknown. Wade and Langton Hewer (1987), after reviewing previous studies, estimate the prevalence to be 1/1000 of the population in the UK. It usually starts in young adult life, occasionally in adolescents or even young children. Very occasionally it occurs for the first time in middle age but rarely after 50. It is a disease of temperate climates, very rare in the Tropics, India or the West Indies. In Australia and South Africa, it is also rare except in the first generation of immigrants from countries frequently affected.

As yet, there is no cure for multiple sclerosis. However a course of adrenocorticotrophic hormone (ACTH) in the acute stages of a relapse will often produce a more rapid and marked improvement than would have been expected naturally. Moreover anti-spastic medication may help flexor spasms and spasticity. Many people with multiple sclerosis turn to alternative treatments in an effort to relieve their symptoms. These range from special diets to the use of hyperbaric oxygen. The effectiveness of such treatments remains unproven.

Motor neurone disease

Motor neurone disease is the name given to a group of related progressive degenerative diseases affecting the motor neurones in the brain and spinal cord. These include progressive muscular atrophy, progressive bulbar palsy and amyotrophic lateral sclerosis (ALS). Confusion reigns over the terminology because in the USA amyotrophic lateral sclerosis is used instead of motor neurone disease and does not have the more specific clinical meaning that ALS has in this country (Cochrane, 1987).

The three forms of motor neurone disease listed above may overlap and merge as the disease progresses. The onset is insidious but the course is relentless. Weakness may first be noticed in the hands, the shoulders or the neck muscles. Hand and shoulder girdle muscles begin to waste and gradually the weakness and wasting spreads throughout the body until the trunk muscles no longer give support (Bickerstaff, 1978). Speech and swallowing of both food and saliva become more difficult as the tongue and throat muscles weaken. Respiratory failure occurs late. Death is usually due to respiratory infection, inhalation pneumonia, respiratory failure or asphyxia.

Amyotrophic lateral sclerosis is the commonest form of motor neurone disease (approximately 66%). It involves both upper and lower motor neurones and is characterized by muscle weakness, spasticity, hyperactive reflexes and emotional liability. It usually starts in the over 55s, and carries on average survival rate, from diagnosis, of 3–4 years. Males are more affected than females (3:2). **Progressive muscular atrophy** affects about 7.5% of patients with motor neurone disease. Lower motor neurone degeneration causes muscle wasting and weakness with loss of weight and fasciculation. Age of onset is usually under 50. Most patients survive more than 5 years after diagnosis. Males are more affected than females (5:1).

Progressive bulbar palsy involves paralysis of the bulbar musculature by a lower motor neurone lesion of the cranial nerves controlling speech and swallowing. Dysphagia and dysarthria progress to the stage where swallowing and speaking are impossible. Alternative means of feeding (by nasogastric tube or gastrostomy) may be necessary as well as the use of communication aids. Progressive bulbar palsy occurs mostly in older people and is slightly more common in women. Survival from onset of symptoms is usually between 6 months and 3 years.

Motor neurone disease affects neither the three cranial nerves which control movement of the eyes nor the lower sacral segments of the spinal cord. The sensory nerves and the autonomic nervous system are also spared. Intellect and memory remain intact throughout. However fatigue, emotional lability, depression, anxiety and insomnia, constipation, pain and discomfort may occur.

Wade and Langton Hewer (1987) assume the following figures for motor neurone disease: an incidence of 2/100 000/ year and a prevalence of 6/100 000. There is no cure. However, treatment of the secondary features listed above may significantly improve the quality of the patient's remaining life.

Further information on motor neurone disease is available in Cochrane (1987) and in the publications of the Motor Neurone Disease Association (from which some of this was taken).

Parkinson's disease

Parkinsonism is a syndrome characterized by tremor of a particular type, muscular rigidity, bradykinesia or hypokinesia
(slowness and poverty of movement) and postural instability.
It can be idiopathic (cause unknown), drug-induced (especially
in those taking a high dosage of tranquillizers), post-encepha-
litic (following some years after an encephalitis) or due to MPTP
toxicity (Caird, 1991).

Symptoms arise from a lack of dopamine in the basal nuclei.
Cells in the substantia nigra degenerate and fail to regulate and
control movement. Any one symptom may predominate. An
initial tremor of the hand may spread to the other hand and
then to the whole body. Classic 'pill-rolling' tremor involves
the thumb and occurs about five times per second. Tremor is
worst when the patient is at rest and increases with emotion.
It improves when he moves and disappears when he is asleep.

Rigidity refers to a resistance to movement. When interrupted
by tremor, it gives a jerky sensation like a cog-wheel (felt by
moving a joint.) Lead-pipe rigidity is felt when the resistance is
about the same throughout the whole range of movement.
Rigidity forces the patient to walk in small shuffling steps,
stooped forwards, arms and legs bent with the arms held across
the body instead of swinging normally. Bradykinesia and hypokinesia prevent him from initiating and performing movements
quickly enough. Thus his movements may be slow and he may
be unable to get out of the chair or turn over in bed. He may
find it difficult to start walking. Once he does, he may be unable
to stop, moving forwards more and more quickly, adopting a
'festinating gait'.

There are two features common in many Parkinsonian
patients. These are known as 'freezing' and 'the on-off phenomenon'. Freezing refers to the sudden inability to complete a
motor activity, for example speaking or walking. It occurs without warning and usually lasts for a few minutes. The 'on-off
phenomenon' refers to a fluctuation in the patient's response to
the levodopa drug: the 'off' period, lasting from minutes to
hours, is when it is ineffective and the 'on' period is when it
works. Postural instability causes the patient to fall. He may
have a 'mask-like' facial appearance due to impaired movement
of the facial musculature. His dysarthric speech is monotonous

and rapidly produced so that at times it may be unintelligible. The autonomic system is also disturbed as shown by excessive formation of saliva, sweating and greasiness of the skin. In the late stages of the disease, dementia is common.

Wade and Langton Hewer (1987) assume the following figures for Parkinson's disease for the UK: an incidence of 18/100 000/year and a prevalence of 160/100 000. The sex incidence is practically equal. Treatment includes the use of drugs, of which there are two principal groups. Dopaminergic drugs, such as levodopa or bromocriptine, enhance or imitate the action of dopamine, while anticholinergic drugs damp down cholinergic activity (involving the neurotransmitter acetylcholine). Physicians have different opinions about the best course of drug treatment but nurses and paramedical staff can also help to alleviate symptoms. Despite treatment, Parkinsonism causes progressive disability with age.

Further information on Parkinson's disease is available in Caird (1991).

Alzheimer's disease

Alzheimer's disease is named after Alois Alzheimer, a German professor of psychiatry in 1906. It is a form of irreversible presenile dementia and is a degenerative disorder affecting the brain. It causes impairment of intellectual functioning. There is a progressive decline in the ability to remember, learn, think and reason. The cause is unknown.

The diagnosis of Alzheimer's disease is one of exclusion because other diseases with a similar clinical picture must be ruled out, for example delirium, paranoid disorders, acute confusional state secondary to infection and drug-induced confusion (Hamdy *et al.*, 1990). Multi-infarct dementia is not the same as Alzheimer's disease. It is abrupt in onset and progresses in a stepwise fashion rather than a steady decline. It is caused by small strokes that are not noticed until many have occurred and sufficient brain tissue has been destroyed, resulting in dementia. Alzheimer's disease is characterized by microscopic changes in the brain, referred to as fibrillary tangles or plaques. Its incidence and prevalence remain obscure. However the Alzheimer's Disease Society estimates the number of sufferers in the UK at about 500 000 (i.e nearly 1% of the population).

The rate at which symptoms occur varies from person to person. Initially these are not always distinguishable from the forgetfulness of depression, bereavement, stress, anxiety, or gradual ageing. There is a loss of short-term memory. The patient becomes disorientated and confused in time and place. As the disease progresses, loss of the ability to think and reason becomes more marked so that tasks such as tying a shoelace or telling the time become impossible.

Gradually all memory is lost, even of words spoken a few minutes before. Speech becomes disordered and incoherent and the patient is unable to look after himself properly. He requires assistance to dress, feed, find his way around the house, maintain personal hygiene and so on. Physically, his condition may remain quite good but his poor mental state and lack of insight place an increasingly heavy burden upon family and friends. Wandering, often at night, and incontinence can be particularly difficult to cope with. There is no cure. The aim is to reduce as many of the consequences of the condition as possible, reducing the stress on caring relatives. The cause of death is often pneumonia or some other type of infection.

Further information on Alzheimer's Disease is available in Hamdy *et al.* (1990).

Cerebral tumours

There are several kinds of cerebral tumours (or neoplasms). General features include raised intracranial pressure, possible hydrocephalus and gradual onset of symptoms (in complete contrast to the sudden onset of stroke). The signs of raised intracranial pressure include headache, vomiting, diplopia, blurring of vision, slowing of the pulse, increasing drowsiness and dilation of the pupils which fail to react to light. However the classic sign is papilloedema – swelling of the optic disc (seen through an ophthalmoscope).

Localized damage to the brain at the site of the tumour may cause fits and/or loss of function directly linked to the area of brain involved; for example there may be paralysis of the opposite side of the body, dysphasia, personality disturbances (if the frontal lobe is affected), ataxia (if the tumour is in the cerebellum), dysphagia (if it affects the cranial nerves of swallowing in the brainstem) and so on.

Fits may affect all parts of the body or be focal fits, affecting only one part (for example the hand). They may not even be full-blown fits but rather alterations in sensation. Tumours in the temporal lobe may cause epilepsy, fragmentary memories and feelings of *déjà vu*. Parietal lobe fits may present as sudden, transient attacks of sensory loss in one limb. Occipital lobe fits may present as flashes of light.

There are different types of cerebral tumour for which the prognosis varies.

1. The Gliomas develop from the glial cells and includes astrocytomas, oligodendrogliomas and glioblastomas. They invade the brain tissue itself, vary in malignancy (depending upon the type of glioma), but the prognosis is poor generally.
2. A haemangioblastoma is a tumour of immature blood vessels usually formed in the cerebellum. It carries a favourable prognosis if there is total excision of both the tumour and its surrounding cyst.
3. A medulloblastoma, usually seen in children under 12, develops from primitive cells in the roof of the IVth ventricle and spreads into the cerebellum and brainstem. It usually recurrs and the prognosis is poor. An ependymoma is another tumour arising in the same area.
4. Acoustic neuromas grow from the sheath of the VIIIth cranial nerve in the cerebello-pontine angle. They are benign but can be completely removed if diagnosed early enough.
5. Pituitary tumours may be one of three kinds (eosiniphil adenoma, basophil adenoma and chromophobe adenoma) depending upon which cells they arise from. They are usually benign.
6. Meningiomas are benign, growing from the arachnoid mater. They can be removed completely.
7. Metastatic tumours are secondary tumours, carried to the nervous system by the blood from a primary tumour elsewhere, for example from the lungs, breast or bowel. There are usually many of them, they develop quickly and are untreatable.

Wade and Langton Hewer (1987), after summarizing previous

studies, estimate an incidence of eight primary and eight secondary tumours per 100 000 of the UK population per year. Little is known about the prevalence of brain tumours or the disability they cause.

Myaesthenia gravis

Myaesthenia gravis is an illness marked by abnormally sudden onset of weakness during sustained or repeated contraction of the muscles. The weakness can be so severe that it causes complete paralysis. After a period of rest, this weakness recovers and responds to anticholinesterase drugs. The illness is caused by an abnormality in the neuromuscular junction. It prevents impulses passing across the point where the finest branches of the motor nerves end in the muscle fibres.

The eye muscles are most frequently affected. Those involved in chewing and swallowing are the next most commonly affected and then the muscles of the face, neck, shoulders, pelvic girdle, limbs and trunk. Symptoms include drooping eyelids, squinting, ptosis, hoarseness, a nasal voice, and difficulties in chewing and swallowing. Classically the muscles become more and more fatigued as an activity progresses. Thus the symptoms are usually more prominent at the end of the day.

The Tensilon Test may be used to confirm the diagnosis. This involves giving the patient, intravenously, 1 ml (10 mg) of eprophonium chloride. This will restore power to normal in one minute. The effect may last for five minutes or longer. Severity of the disease fluctuates and long periods of remission may occur. Relapses may be caused by infection, trauma or psychological stress. Wade and Langton Hewer (1987) estimate the incidence in the UK to be four per million and the prevalence to be 40 per million. Treatment involves the use of drugs (neostigmine and pyridostigmine) but the dose is crucial. An overdose causes the patient to become increasingly weak and not to respond to his drugs.

Guillain-Barré syndrome

Guillain-Barré syndrome is an acute distress of the nervous system involving the spinal nerve roots, peripheral nerves and cranial nerves. It is characterized by polyneuritis, or inflammation of the nerves, following a viral infection. The disease can affect either sex at any age. The acute phase of this lower motor neurone lesion involves rapid onset of paralysis of the limbs along with sensory loss and muscle atrophy. The initial illness, followed by flaccid paralysis, may affect all four limbs at once or may begin in the legs and spread upward to the arms. It may involve the muscles of respiration. The disease is thought to be due to a disordered immune response. Neurological symptoms are sometimes preceded by a mild flu-like illness.

Wade and Langton Hewer (1987) state that an average Health District in the UK (comprising a population of 250 000 people) may have two or three cases of Guillain-Barré syndrome a year and will need to ventilate one every other year. They add that many mild cases may remain undiagnosed and not be referred to hospital. Prognosis is varied and improvement may be sporadic. Almost complete recovery may be gained within 3 – 6 months or more. However recovery may be incomplete with slight remissions, serious relapses or plateauing.

Huntingdon's chorea

Huntingdon's chorea is a chronic progressive inherited disease for which there is no cure. It is characterized pathologically by degeneration of the ganglion cells of the forebrain and corpus striatum. It affects both men and women. The age of onset of symptoms is usally 30–45 but it may be either later or earlier. Those which appear first are choreic movements and these develop insidiously. As the disorder progresses, it leads to dysarthria and ataxia of the upper limbs and of the gait. Mental changes gradually develop, usually a few years after the onset of the chorea and there is progressive dementia. In most cases, Huntingdon's chorea is progressive and terminates fatally, usually within 10–15 years of onset. However the duration of the disease varies and the drugs reserpine or tetrabenazine may help to reduce the chorea.

Wade and Langton Hewer's (1987) review gives the prevalence of the disease in the UK as varying between 2.5 and 9.2/ 100 000.

Friedreich's ataxia

This is a hereditary disease involving degeneration of the spinal cord which is unusually small. The heart, too, shows diffuse change. It is enlarged due to thickening of the muscle and diffuse fibrosis. The age of onset, that is, when the patient first appears with the symptom, is between 5 and 15 years. These symptoms include ataxic gait and, later on, ataxic movement in the upper limbs and intention tremor. In the later stages, speech is dysarthric. Most cases show nystagmus and weakness due to corticospinal tract degeneration as well as pes cavus and scoliosis. Cardiac changes can lead to heart failure. The disease is slow but progressive. Few patients live for more than 20 years after the onset of symptoms. The estimated prevalence of the disease in the UK is 2/100 000 (Wade and Langton Hewer, 1987).

Meningitis and encephalitis

Meningitis is an inflammation of the membranous coverings of the brain and spinal cord. There are three main types. **Pyogenic meningitis** is caused by pus-forming bacteria (for example meningococci, pneumococci and the influenza bacillus). **Tuberculous meningitis** is caused by the tubercle bacillus. **Viral meningitis** develops from a number of different viruses, for example the polio virus and the mumps virus. Symptoms of meningitis include an initial few days of flu-like signs, high temperature and a cold or sore throat. Headache then develops rapidly, spreading backwards, causing neck and back pain. Vomiting and photophobia occur as well followed by drowsiness, restlessness, irritability and – classically – neck stiffness or rigidity. Kernig's sign is positive. A lumbar puncture is used to confirm meningitis. This allows the cerbrospinal fluid to be studied. Pyogenic and tuberculous meningitis are treated with drugs. However viral meningitis is not definitely affected by these.

Encephalitis refers to inflammation of the brain. It may be due to bacteria (from infected sinuses, ears and so on), or to viruses (for example the herpes simplex virus) or, in some countries, to parasites acquired from animals. General features include moderate headache, vomiting, confusion, delirium and increasing drowsiness which develops into coma and epileptic fits. There is little neck stiffness (unless the illness is meningoencephalitic, where the meninges are involved as well). Kernig's sign is negative. Encephalitis caused by bacteria may develop into a brain abscess which requires surgery and drug treatment. Viral encephalitis may be treated by steroids early on.

Wade and Langton Hewer (1987) state that viral encephalitis and meningitis may have an annual incidence in the UK of 7.4 to 10.9 per 100 000 respectively. Bacterial meningitis may have an incidence of 9.5/100 000/year. They add that the average Health District may therefore face about 70 patients requiring admission for diagnosis of meningitis or encephalitis each year, each staying at least 1 week and being seen once. An occasional patient will be left severely disabled by herpes simplex encephalitis or bacterial meningitis.

2

Patients' and relatives' views

SELF-HELP GROUPS

There are several societies devoted to helping the neurologically damaged adult and his family, both in the US and in the UK. Many have evolved out of sheer frustration and desperation. The patient and his relatives have often felt that they were not getting the help they really wanted. Some complain that their voice has been ignored. Others add that health professionals neither understand the true nature of their problems nor empathize with their situation. Accordingly, individuals with direct practical experience of neurological illness have been driven to form various self-help groups.

An example of this is The Parkinson's Disease Society. This was founded in 1969 by Miss Mali Jenkins (1904–1989) whose sister, Sarah, had Parkinson's Disease. She discovered that no society existed to help people with the disease or their families. She knew, from experience, that there was a desperate need for greater public understanding and support. With Eryl, her sister, she founded a society from a bedroom in her house. Initially, it aimed to provide information but the services expanded as the demand grew (Baker and McCall, 1991).

The Alzheimer's Disease Society also grew out of direct personal experience. Cora Phillips, a retired nurse, had to look after her husband for 10 years, before he eventually died of Alzheimer's disease, aged 68. These were years of suffering and tragedy for both Mr Phillips and his family. After meeting other families with the same problems, Mrs Phillips saw the need for shared knowledge, mutual help, understanding and support. Accordingly she helped to set up the Alzheimer's Disease Society.

The societies or associations in the UK which cater for the adult with acquired neurological damage include the following groups:

- The Stroke Association. Launched in November 1991, this developed from The Chest, Heart and Stroke Association (CHSA). From now on, the stroke work of the CHSA is continued and enhanced in the new Stroke Association while the chest and heart side has been handed over to other major charities specializing in these areas. (The change of name does not apply to the Scotland Chest, Heart and Stroke Association or the Northern Ireland Chest, Heart and Stroke Association.)
- Headway, a society devoted to the needs of the head injured and his family.
- The Multiple Sclerosis Society of Great Britain and Northern Ireland.
- The Motor Neurone Disease Association (MNDA).
- The Parkinson's Disease Society.
- The Alzheimer's Disease Society.
- The Myasthenia Gravis Association.
- The Guillain–Barré Syndrome Support Group.
- The Huntingdon's Disease Association.
- The Friedreich's Ataxia Group.

Similar societies exist in the US. These include the following groups:

- Stroke Clubs International.
- The National Head Injury Foundation, Inc.
- The National Multiple Sclerosis Society.
- The American Parkinson Disease Association.
- The Parkinson's Disease Foundation.

Numerous others exist as well.

FEATURES COMMON TO ALL GROUPS

Each society or association is concerned exclusively with a specific type of neurological impairment. Their focus of interest is reflected in their titles. However analysis of a range of the publications, of all of the groups listed above, reveals certain common trends. These are discussed below.

Similar aims and functions

First of all, they appear to have similar aims and functions. Broadly speaking each organization tries to:

1. raise public awareness of the disease it covers;
2. provide information about it. This may range from a summary of the basic symptoms and recognized treatment procedures to reports on recent research and on aids and resources;
3. encourage the provision of adequate services;
4. act as a link for families and friends via support groups;
5. fund research into the disorder;
6. provide newsletters. These cover topics ranging from practical help and advice, to news about member patients and their relatives. There is also discussion about fund-raising activities, research trends, new publications, and other relevant issues.

Recurrent themes

Another similarity links the self-help groups listed above. Their various newsletters, leaflets and publications contain several common themes. Time and again, the same topics recur, although they may be couched in different words. The rest of this chapter lists these topics and discusses them in further detail.

1. Ignorance

Generally speaking, patients and their families were normal people going about their daily business before the illness took hold. A vast range of activities might have occupied their lives. Work, holidays, sport, family commitments and friendships are just a few examples. The majority of such people, at this stage, have limited knowledge, if any, of neurological disease. They may have heard vaguely of illnesses such as multiple sclerosis or Parkinson's disease. They may even know of somebody who, for example, has had a stroke. Television and the media may have highlighted certain conditions; for example the death of David Niven, a well-known actor, boosted the publicity surrounding motor neurone disease. However most people will be unfamiliar with the causes, symptoms and prognoses of different neurological conditions – let alone the burden which these often entail for the patient's family.

Accordingly, a sudden head injury or diagnosis of a cerebral tumour comes as a total shock. Patient and family may feel completely ignorant about the medical world which now engulfs them. Eric writes about this when told his wife had MS.

'I knew nothing about MS. I didn't even know what it was.'
Multiple Sclerosis Society, 1990.

This feeling may be as acute for sombody diagnosed at home in the community as it is for the patient who has been admitted to hospital. Ignorance due to scarcity of information is a common complaint. A relative of someone with Alzheimer's disease writes

'I received absolutely no informational support. I stumbled onto what I needed accidentally, and who knows what support was available that I never did hear of.'
Somners and Zarit, 1985, p. 30.

Talbott (1989, p. 3) reinforces this view. He states that in hospitals where an individual has been admitted with a head injury, information is scarce. '. . . the most common early complaint of relatives is that they are told nothing and can find no one to ask.'

The situation is not helped by the uniforms which staff wear. Professionals' statuses and jobs are unclear because, to the uninitiated, everyone seems to be dressed the same. The doctor and the speech and language therapist may both wear a white coat. Of course their name badges may proclaim their identity but relatives do not tend to scrutinize these at first meeting, particularly when they are desperate to talk face-to-face with someone. In any case, even hospital staff can make mistakes about the identity of the person standing by the beside in a white coat. Similarly the student nurse and the staff may wear identical dresses. Again, the significance of different epaulettes or hat-stripe colour is lost to one who has never been in a hospital before. The situation is comparable to a visit to an army barracks by someone who knows nothing about rank and its relationship with hats or ribbons.

Scarcity of information is compounded by the use of medical

jargon and unfamiliar, intimidating, highly technical life-saving equipment. The MNDA newsletter (Spring 1990) stresses the need to provide patients and their families with information – and this goes for any kind of progressive condition, not just motor neurone disease. Family caring for a relative at home in the community can feel equally ignorant.

2. Problems on discharge

Professional texts recognize that discharge home into the community is a crucial event for both the patient and his family. 'All the care shared by a hospital staff team now falls on one or two family members' (Talbott, 1989, p. 6). With this in mind, any competent therapist will arrange ongoing support. Attendance at a day hospital, use of a home help, regular respite care in hospital every 8 weeks or so, and domiciliary therapy are just a few of the possibilities (Garner, 1990). Nevertheless all parties know that the buck now stops at home. Hospitalization may have provided invaluable physical and psychological space (for both patient and family) but this now disappears. It is the family who must now face up to carrying the load.

Discharge, therefore, can come as a real shock. 'No matter how much work you put into preparing the relatives for the patient's discharge, it is almost certain that they will never be ready' (Garner, 1990, p. 105). This experience often produces resentment and bitterness. Relatives who have appeared aimiable and supportive during hospital visits may turn against the very professionals who think they are helping. They may become demanding and critical under the growing burden of care (Lees, 1988).

Complaints are voiced in the literature – 'I feel that the professionals involved in Sheila's care at the time could have listened more to our ideas and suggestions' (Multiple Sclerosis Society, 1990, Chapter 3, p. 3). They also surface informally at meetings of individual self-help groups.

Here is an example which occurred at a local Headway meeting. A 17-year-old youth received severe head injuries following a motor cycle crash in town. Regular physiotherapy for several months ensured that he was at least able to walk when he went home, albeit with an abnormal gait. By about 2 years after discharge, his physical recovery had plateaued. However the physiotherapist maintained contact with the patient and his family by arranging 6-monthly reviews and by attending the local Headway meetings. Over time, they began to complain bitterly about the lack of regular physiotherapy. They maintained this should involve regular sessions using an exercise bike. They claimed this would further improve the patient's gait. The physiotherapist felt this was unlikely given several factors, including the severity of his injuries, the amount of physiotherapy he had already received, his response to this and the time which had elapsed since the accident. Despite sympathetic and diplomatic discussion on her part, patient and family remained adamant. The physiotherapist received strong personal criticism, verging on allegations of negligence.

This example highlights the difficulties which may arise in the community, weeks, months and even years after discharge. Emotional and psychological factors may be the root cause; for example, frustration and anger at a lifestyle which has been lost. However they may be expressed through physical means. Lees (1988) gives thoughtful consideration to the social and emotional consequences of severe brain injury in the light of her own experience and recent research (Weddell et al., 1980; Brooks, 1984; Brooks et al. 1986; Livingstone, 1986a, 1986b). Indeed 'one has only to go to any Headway meeting to realize that the problems are generally only just beginning when the patient is discharged' (Garner, 1990, p. 129).

3. Isolation and hopelessness

Isolation and hopelessness are feelings which recur frequently in the literature and newsletters of the various self-help groups. Patients write about their own isolation as they struggle to function at home in the community. To Stephen Pegg, motor neurone disease is a state of being 'locked in solitary confinement . . . as each muscle in my body mutinies against the orders sent out by my brain' (Pegg, 1989–90, p. 10). For Michel Monnot, Parkinson's Disease is a devastating illness '. . . leaving me speechless, mouth agape, clutching at receding threads of memory which vanish into the fog of my muted and engulfing solitude' (Monnot, 1988, p. 1).

Relatives and carers suffer as well. They use the newsletters as a way of sharing their sense of isolation, thereby reaching out to others in the same situation. Mrs K. J. Scott, in an article entitled 'Bereavement Without a Burial', describes the loneliness of caring for her husband with Alzheimer's disease. 'You feel there is no way of coping: nobody cares, you are on your own 24 hours a day, with no light at the end of a long and very dark tunnel' (Alzheimer's Disease Society Newsletter, November 1990, p. 3).

Friendships slowly disintegrate as relationships alter irrevocably. Mrs P. J. describes the loneliness of her head-injured son. 'No, his mates don't seem to come round any more. Well, he's not the same, is he?' (Headway Newsletter, 14 March 1990). His enforced solitude tears her apart as she remembers the sociable fun-loving son she has lost.

Sometimes carers impose their isolation upon themselves deliberately. By struggling on and coping alone, they avoid the guilt they know they will feel when they admit that they need help. Eric reflects on this as he contemplates accepting professional help at home for his wife with MS.

Asking for outside help comes only after years of coping alone. Inevitably by this time the carer is tired, anxious about the future and feels trapped unable to make any plans on a daily basis or in the future. Hopefully outside help will be welcomed but human nature being what it is, it may also be slightly resented: by the carer who has to admit that he or she is unable to cope; by the person with MS whose privacy is invaded.

Multiple Sclerosis Society, 1990

The MNDA literature emphasizes the problems which may arise in the community when too many professionals are involved at once. Bombarding the family with visits and advice leads to loss of privacy and autonomy. The authors advocate sharing and overlapping of team roles to cut down on unnecessary visits. In some districts a 'key worker' is responsible for liaising with the family and coordinating help at the appropriate times. This should be a person of any discipline to whom the family relates well, who is accessible and aware of all the other services available.

Feelings of isolation and hopelessness may lead to anger and violence. The American Parkinson's Disease Association highlights the plight of adult children as carers, particularly daughters. All too often they are physically and emotionally overburdened with the many roles they have to play. They are daughter and nurse to the patient, supporter and counsellor to their other parents, as well as mother to their own children and wife to their husband. Hamdy *et al.* (1990) refer to the 'sandwich generation' when discussing the carers of those with Alzheimer's disease. They use the term to refer to individuals who must care for both children and elderly people with dementia. Bathing and help with basic daily functions is required for both groups.

Multirole demands create more pressure and build up stress levels. It is no surprise to hear of cases of violence in these situations. Tragically, this may be violence against the patient – whom the carer loves and whose suffering she is desperate to alleviate. Violence may occur in an over-protective, claustrophobic relationship completely out of the blue. Usually at this stage, tensions have built up to a critical level and the last straw has broken the camels's back (Multiple Sclerosis Society, 1990).

4. Optimism

However the negative themes of ignorance, isolation, hopelessness and violence are not the only topics to surface in the literature. Positive aspects also recur. One of these is optimism – often appearing against apparently insurmountable odds. Robinson describes the fighting spirit, borne of desperation, which confronts the progressive neurological decline of motor neurone disease.

> Many of us have seen the health of a previously robust member of our family decline rapidly and go beyond the point of recovery. We want answers as quickly as possible, and to help in any way we can to obtain them.
>
> Robinson, 1990, p. 2

It is this desperate optimism which often confronts the professional, particularly if the patient has been referred to her late on in the course of his disease. Relatives are not concerned with how many cases of terminal neurological illness she has treated previously. They want action here and now. It is their mother, father, child or relative who is dying. One way of empathizing with the family is for the professional to put herself in their situation and imagine how they feel. This may influence how she responds to their demands which may seem to be hopeless and unrealistic at times.

Optimism even surfaces in those coping with the progressive dementia of Alzheimer's disease. Mrs K. J. Scott does not dwell on her feelings of isolation and hopelessness as described above. She fights on. 'I won't give up on him. While there is a little bit left alive in his brain, I will push to try and keep a bit of him still there' (Scott, 1990, p. 3).

Other optimistic comments come from patients themselves. Suzanne Rogers in the US was diagnosed as having multiple sclerosis 20 years ago. Yet she still manages to convey some practical thoughts in her pamphlet for those who have been newly diagnosed. 'Believe it or not though, some very positive growth can come from all this' (Rogers, 1990, p. 2). Her text is full of positive advice delivered in non-threatening, everyday language which is easy to understand. She recommends, for example, that the person should find a doctor with whom they can talk easily. (Fortunately, changing GPs has become much easier in the UK with recent government health legislation).

Other suggestions include accessing helpful and hopeful literature, controlling weight gain by following slowly a sensible diet, planning activities for enjoyment rather than necessity, finding a supportive physical therapist and so on. An encouraging, optimistic note permeates her booklet. This is what patients and their relatives want and need to hear – if their remarks in their various newsletters are anything to go by. They do not appreciate obscure, unfamiliar medical and academic jargon which describes their condition but fails to give them any hope or practical advice.

The newsletters contain examples of patients triumphing in the face of adversity. Although multiple sclerosis forced William Pennington to leave his job, he did not give up. He continued to organize the Huntsville, Tennessee volunteer fire department and was elected fire chief. The professional may view such *ad hoc*, 'lay' accounts as anecdotal trimming. She may favour professional texts which assume a thorough knowledge and understanding of the neurological disability involved. However anecdotal and personal accounts are often the very things that keep the patient going and provide motivation for cooperation with therapy.

5. Promotional and fund raising activities

News about promotional and fund raising activities are a further major component of the self-help group literature. Sponsored swims and walks, open days and raffles abound. Again to the patient and his family, these may be highly important events. Professionals may be approached to lend their support. The temptation may be to avoid getting involved and to concentrate on the nuts and bolts of professional treatment. However, positive social activities may generate more enthusiasm in both patient and family than professional treatment activities. They may prefer to concentrate on assisting the financial and scientific effort surrounding attempts to find a cure for the disease.

6. Broad coverage of research

Most societies follow closely the latest research developments surrounding their disease. The Multiple Sclerosis Society summarizes the alternative treatments which are available. These range from special diets (for example the use of sunflower seed oil and evening primrose oil) to hyperbaric oxygen and allergy-related treatment. The society keeps up to date with current research activities and offers members a fair assessment of their effectiveness.

Similarly, the Alzheimer's Disease Society keeps abreast of research into, for example, abnormal protein synthesis and its effect on brain cells, environmental variables such as nutrition and absorption of metals, viruses and the role of the body's immune system, the potential for fetal brain transplants and so on. The MNDA newsletters carry regular reports on research news; for example the Spring 1990 issue summarized investigations surrounding 'POMC neuropeptides in regenerating motor neurones' and 'Transfer of toxins between motor neurones: a possible mechanism of motor neuronal death in MND'. Their reports are concise. They can be understood without a medical qualification or experience of working in the health professions.

Another example is the Stroke Association which provides accessible information on stroke. Pamphlets include one giving 20 questions and answers about stroke and reducing its risk. The Parkinson's Disease Foundation summarizes, amongst other topics, the latest findings on intracerebral transplantation in the treatment of Parkinson's Disease and the use of the anti-epileptic drug clonazepam in the treatment of Parkinsonian dysarthria. Many societies have used professional help in formulating their pamphlets. Doctors, nurses and paramedics have provided information using their professional expertise.

7. Practical information and help

One of the major benefits of the self-help group literature is the wealth of practical information and advice it contains. In my experience there is no comparable source which describes, as concisely, what the patient needs to know. For this reason the information should be essential reading for professionals – particularly if they want to learn about all the aspects of the patient's illness.

Pamphlets contain practical suggestions by the score on how to cope with problems caused by the disease; for example the 'MNDA Fact Sheet for Patient and Carer No. 1' lists the clothing available for those who dribble or cannot swallow their saliva. Many professionals may find this information useful for their patients with motor neurone disease, Parkinson's disease and multiple sclerosis, for example. Careful choice of clothing can greatly improve comfort and make the problem much less noticeable. The fact sheet illustrates dress and jumper styles which disguise wet areas. However in my experience neither professional training nor academic texts stress important management tips like these. Teaching concentrates more on assessment and treatment.

Similarly, the literature on multiple sclerosis covers topics as varied as 'What is MS?', 'Help From Local Authorities', 'Getting the Best out of Telephone, Gas, Electricity, Water', 'Multiple Sclerosis: the Case for Telling the Truth', and many others. The information pack for professional carers includes everything the individual should know – including advice on pregnancy, parenthood and contraception. Therapists can learn a huge amount from reading these booklets and pamphlets. They include more information than that supplied in the traditional, academic and teaching texts. Thus they help the therapist to appreciate the global needs of the patient and his family. Relevant advertising provides an additional, useful source of information.

Indeed some pamphlets and booklets are aimed specifically at professionals. The MNDA and The Multiple Sclerosis Society of Great Britain and Northern Ireland are just two associations which provide this type of information. The therapist who reads these will recognize aspects of her own treatment but will learn much more about that provided by other professionals. This gives her a sound base for understanding what the others are trying to achieve.

Sharing of information like this is vital for the sake of the patient.

> Very often poor communication between different professionals, and between hospital and community services, left us worrying whether or not support would be available when needed.
>
> Multiple Sclerosis Society, 1990, section 3

Reading the self-help group literature gives the therapist a head start in understanding the activities of other professionals. This makes it easier for her to decide when to call them in – a vital skill in providing efficient team care.

> . . . there should always be a blurring of professional boundaries. However, it is important for all professionals to know what their limitations are and when to call in their colleagues.
>
> Motor Neurone Disease Association.

8. Depth of knowledge of disease

Another theme stands out in the self-help group literature. This is the depth of knowledge of the disease shown by both patient and family and their involvement in it. Banks (1990), discussing multiple sclerosis, says that patients often know a lot more than nurses and junior doctors. Expertise is not uniquely acquired through professional training. Patients are also experts, with a different kind of expertise gained from direct experience.

The following remarks, taken from the literature, reflect patients' knowledge of both the physical and mental characteristics of their disease and its treatment.

Not only must physical care be given – the mind, the 'self'

need care, too and both kinds of care must begin as soon as the stroke person returns home from hospital

Morton, 1990b, p. 5

My experience has proved that there is a lot more to head injury than the repair of the physical damage. Although to all intents and purposes outwardly I appear fully recovered and 'normal', I still have considerable mental problems and am unable to return to work . . . I am unable to talk to somebody on the telephone and write a message down at the same time . . . I am subject to violent outbursts. Life is now completely changed

Anon, 1990, p. 4

I didn't want people's sympathy but I wanted them to understand

Multiple Sclerosis Society, 1990, Vol. 3, p. 3

SIGNIFICANCE FOR THE PROFESSIONAL

The sections above cover a range of topics found in the self-help group literature. These have implications for the professional at work both in hospital and in the community. The most obvious is to read a selection of the various pamphlets and newsletters, if only to obtain practical information about a particular neurological disease and its current state of research. Many therapists may have the information already. However revision itself can prove a useful exercise, highlighting various points which might otherwise have been forgotten.

A further advantage, however, is to gain an insight into (or remember again) how the illness may affect patients and their families. Their feelings and opinions will influence their response to therapy and therefore the success of any proposed treatment and management. Thus even the best-laid plans may go awry – which can be frustrating, particularly for the student and newly or recently qualified therapist. Eager to show relatives ways of helping the patient, she may expend vast amounts of enthusiasm, energy and time; for example the physiotherapist may wish to demonstrate the best way of positioning and handling; the occupational therapist may be desperate to share information about appropriate dressing techniques; and the speech and language therapist may want the relatives to use a communication aid (such as a 'Lightwriter') as a supplement to speech.

All such well-founded plans may founder, however, in the face of reluctance and lack of cooperation. Relatives may fail to attend appointments on the ward or be unavailable in the home during the domiciliary visit. They may not put the advice they have been given into practice. This can be very frustrating for those involved in treatment. Poor patient progress can be blamed on apparently obstructive, difficult relatives.

Nevertheless, this behaviour may stem from exactly those concerns voiced in the self-help group literature (and in some professional articles and texts). Those at home may feel that the caring role is theirs alone and that accepting help is an admission of defeat. Or the stress of looking after their sick relatives may be too much. In these cases, alleviating emotional and psychosocial problems may be more important than training the carers. The psychologist or the social worker may have more to offer at this stage. The priorities may alter later on if the relatives are more willing to accept the therapists' help – although in some cases the situation may never change.

A mismatch of priorities may exist not only between patient, relative and therapist but between professionals themselves. Malzer (1988) notes that professionals often fail to agree on a patient's performance. Nurses, physiotherapists, occupational therapists and patients differed considerably in their assessments of patients' functional abilities. Malzer suggests that nurses tend to judge patients as more dependent whereas therapists are attuned to finer nuances in capabilities. Whatever the reason, if even the staff involved in treatment cannot agree, it is no surprise to find that relatives dispute what is done. To cater for this, the therapist may have to modify her treatment aims – even if this means that the patient does not achieve what he is capable of.

The emotional, and psychosocial difficulties expressed in the self-help group literature have a further implication for the professional. As well as reading newsletters and so on, she may want to get involved with the society itself. This is a good way of empathizing with the patient, even if the contact is only superficial. Garner (1990) advocates attending the local Headway group to gain further knowledge of head injury. She maintains that this will give the professional greater understanding and therefore empathy into the family dynamics following head injury.

Indeed putting the patient and family in touch with the self-help group may be beneficial. Therapists may be reluctant to do this. They may place little importance on the literature or the activities of the society for a variety of reasons. They may feel that the information is invalid because it is anecdotal and the writers are not trained professionals; or they may even feel slightly threatened because the society's advice encroaches on their own area of expertise. It is important to avoid this attitude if the patient and family are to come first in health care. Professional territorial behaviour merely limits the possibilities for helping the patient. Indeed relatives are often in the best position to appreciate the predicament of the patient.

One final point about the self-help group literature deserves mention. As seen above, it is full of feelings and intuitions. Unfortunately, Western medicine fails to stress the importance of subjective knowledge like this. It concentrates instead on rational knowledge, objectivity and quantification. East Asian society, on the other hand, places high value on subjective knowledge. Indeed even Japan, with all its high-tech equipment and scientific progress, considers subjective knowledge to be as important as rational deductive thinking (Capra, 1982).

This discrepancy has implications for those professionals working in the West. Despite calls to prove the scientific efficacy of their treatment, therapists should not lose sight of the importance of feelings and intuitions – both their own and those of the people they treat. It is vital to remember that 'beneath the symptoms beats the being of a vulnerable, traumatized person fighting to survive' (Maloney *et al.*, 1985, p. xxi).

Why do patients' experiences fail to figure significantly in the medical literature? Isaacs (1982), a doctor, admits he cannot provide an answer but he does recognize the importance of this kind of information. He describes his efforts to report the intensity and diversity of patients' suffering at home on discharge from hospital following a stroke. He wanted to publish his findings in a medical journal for his medical colleagues. However, ruined lives, destroyed marriages, broken families, bizarre and altered behaviour, bewilderment and perplexity proved to be too 'soft' a material. They were unacceptable for publication.

He eventually did publish a report but after doing a nice hardening job, with scales and tables. However he felt that the vital subjective essence of his study was lost.

His experiences suggest that topics in the self-help group literature (such as those in this chapter) may remain inaccessible to many who work in medicine and its related field. They are simply not considered scientific enough. Yet they provide a vital forum for discussion. In addition they are an important source of information which all therapists may find useful.

CONCLUSION

This chapter has looked at common features in the literature of self-help groups run by, and for, neurologically brain damaged adults and their families. Similar aims and functions figure prominently as well as many recurrent themes. These include patients' and relatives' initial ignorance of the disease and the problems they experience on discharge from hospital. Their feelings of isolation and hopelessness also surface frequently, although a sense of optimism survives in some.

Additional recurrent themes in the literature include news about promotional and fund-raising activities, broad coverage of recent research into the disease, and practical information and help. The literature highlights, furthermore, the detailed level of knowledge often acquired by those who have been affected by a specific neurological illness.

These findings have implications for the professional with regard to teamwork. They highlight the importance of the patient and his relatives within the team. Their roles and experiences are crucial. Acknowledging these and catering for their feelings will influence their attitudes, thereby affecting the success of intervention. Indeed reading the literature of the self-help groups may promote the status of the patient and family within the team by illustrating for the professional their main worries and concerns. These may not necessarily surface during face-to-face encounters. Pamphlets and newsletters also provide a means of revising the facts of a specific neurological condition and learning more about it from the patient's point of view. The final part of this chapter stresses for professionals the relevance and importance of subjective, intuitional knowledge as opposed to objective quantitative data often demanded by the medical world. This is particularly important for successful teamwork which often depends upon the individual's regard for how the patient and his family actually feel rather than knowledge of impersonal numerical facts.

3

The professions

Generally speaking, anyone who enters medicine, nursing, physiotherapy, occupational therapy, speech and language therapy, social work, clinical psychology and so forth does so because they want to practise that profession. As students they will have little, if any, experience of the work of the other professions. The main knowledge they gain about each other will probably be gathered after they have qualified while working in the job.

Successful teamwork depends upon effective communication between the team members involved. This may fail for a variety of reasons, raised frequently in other texts. Personality conflict, staff shortage (and flux), limited opportunities for contact (due to distant locations and incompatible work schedules), the opposition of administration, and disagreement about professional boundaries are just a few of the points which have been discussed (Edwards and Hanley, 1989). Barber and Kratz (1980) stress how difficult it can be to understand the role of a fellow professional. They argue that disciplines are in a continual state of change. They cannot be understood without reference to their historical background.

Most agree, however, that lack of understanding about each others' roles seems to be a major factor, contributing to the problem. It follows, therefore, that learning about each other's professions will assist teamwork (Smyth, 1990) because individual members may begin to appreciate exactly WHY someone chooses to work in a particular way.

Consider the nurse who is taught to be responsible for ensuring that her patient gets enough to eat. Faced with someone who eats slowly, she may give verbal encouragement during the meal – for example 'here's another spoonful', 'would you

like some potato?' and so on. The speech and language therapist, on the other hand, may decide that conversation is distract-
ing the patient. She may feel he needs to concentrate exclusively
on triggering a swallow reflex (which is impaired by his neurological condition). Accordingly she may write in the medical
notes, perhaps even in the nursing Kardex, such advice as 'Do
not talk to the patient whilst he is eating.'

The nurse may choose to ignore this for several reasons. She
may have been off-duty at the time the therapist (who may
work part-time) saw the patient. Furthermore she may not agree
with the advice because the therapist has not explained the
problem fully to her. She may feel unhappy about feeding
someone without talking to them because this contradicts both
her training and natural instinct to communicate with her
patient and encourage him. She may even be unaware that
anything has been written about the patient's swallowing ability
in the nursing Kardex.

The speech and language therapist, on the other hand, may
wonder why her advice is ignored. She may feel threatened by,
and resentful of, the nursing staff. Thus she may shorten her
already infrequent visits to the ward – compounding further
the breakdown in communication, which is deteriorating
rapidly. Once again it is the patient who falls between the
cracks.

One way of assisting teamwork would be to learn about
fellow professions as a student. Admittedly, courses are probably already crammed with the basic professional teaching
essential to carrying out the job. Nevertheless, a word or two
about the others, or even an established reference which could
be consulted at a later date when required, might prove advan-
tageous to those who find themselves entering team care.

This chapter tries to meet this need, albeit briefly. It summarizes the history of those professions which may be involved in
care of the neurologically damaged adult. Those discussed
include doctors, nurses, paramedical staff (both hospital and
community workers), paramedical helpers or assistants, dieticians, social workers and clinical psychologists. Following this,
there is discussion of the pressures which may exert themselves
upon various members of the team.

PROFESSIONAL HISTORIES

Several authors describe at length the history and development of various health professions. The following summary is based on accounts by Richards (1989), Hewlett (1990), Clarke (1991) and Levitt and Wall (1992). It should highlight how specific professions have developed, placing each one within its historical context. Some of the professions, discussed (namely, physiotherapy, occupational therapy, and dietetics) belong to the Council for Professions Supplementary to Medicine (CPSM). This is a statutory body set up under the Professions Supplementary to Medicine Act, 1960. It covers seven specific professions, each represented by a board. It regulates education and training and controls the quality of that training and of the professional qualifications granted. The other professions discussed have different bodies which perform this function.

Medicine

In the UK before 1700, the medical profession consisted of physicians, surgeons and apothecaries. The physicians had the highest status. Their power contributed to the founding of the Royal College of Physicians of London in 1518. Members were Oxbridge graduates who had a religious and classical education. Most of them had also studied medical subjects in European universities. Surgeons, on the other hand, were craftsmen organized in a guild which was associated with the barbers. They were licensed to perform a small range of procedures on unanaesthetized patients. The third group, the apothecaries, were tradesmen. From 1617 they were licensed by the Society of Apothecaries to sell drugs prescribed by physicians.

1745 saw the foundation of the Company of Surgeons. This was independent from the barbers and allowed educational standards to improve. By 1800 the company had become the Royal College of Surgeons of England. Apothecaries also developed in their own right. They became 'general practitioners' in 1703 when they were entitled to see patients and prescribe medicines themselves. In 1815 the Apothecaries Act gave the Society of Apothecaries the right to license those who had served a 5-year apprenticeship and passed exams.

Modern day hospitals, meanwhile, developed from a mixture

of sources. Firstly in the early nineteenth century there were the parish workhouses. These had sick wards where the able-bodied inmates could be treated when they became ill. In addition to these, voluntary hospitals developed. Built and financed through donations and subscriptions from the philan-thropic and the well-to-do, they attracted the services of skilled doctors. Together with the isolation hospitals and the asylums, the workhouses and the voluntary hospitals acted as a public hospital care service.

As time went on, voluntary hospitals came to rely on the services of the Royal Colleges. They no longer recognized the apothecaries who thus became the general practitioners for the middle classes and the poor. This established the distinction between consultants and general practitioners.

The General Medical Council is the body which maintains a register of practitioners and supervises the educational stan-dards of training institutions. The British Medical Association, on the other hand, acts as spokesman for all doctors – both in hospital and general practice. An accident of history accounts for the difference between the titles of 'Dr' and 'Mr' in medicine. Physicians, that is, doctors practising medicine, not surgery, are called 'Dr' while surgeons pride themselves on being called 'Mr'. Both have the same MB University qualification which entitles them to the courtesy title of 'Dr'. Richards (1989) explains that the 'Mr' convention is a form of inverted snobbery. For centuries physicians, with their universtiy education, looked down on surgeons who, as craftsmen, were not accepted as members of a learned profession. In the last century, as described above, surgery became accepted as a full part of medi-cine in its widest sense. Hence the same basic medical qualifi-cations became necessary for physicians and surgeons. Never-theless surgeons proudly retained the title of 'Mr' and have done so ever since. Scottish surgeons, however, prefer to be called 'Dr'.

Nursing

In early civilizations, general nursing care was carried out by women of the household or by slaves rather than by specially trained attendants. Later on, Christianity prompted the devel-opment of the nursing profession as we know it today. The teachings of Christ inspired the early Christians to seek out those needing help. They travelled beyond the narrow limits of their own homes and ministered to the bodily and spiritual needs of the sick and poor. The Order of Deaconesses was formed and worked with the Deacons under the Bishops to become the first organized visiting service.

The medieval period saw further development of the nursing profession. The impetus for this lay with the Church which held great power. Religious orders were responsible for the care of all who needed help, whether from sickness, poverty or old age. Thus in the UK, hospital nursing began as a vocation associated with the monks and nuns of these religious orders at about the same time as hospitals such as St Bartholomews' (1123) and St Thomas' (1215) were founded. The status of the profession, however, was not high. Nursing was considered a sordid duty fit only for 'broken down and drunk old widows' (Carr-Saunders and Wilson, 1933, p. 118). Fortunately, attitudes changed after the mid-nineteenth century.

In 1840 Elizabeth Fry founded an 'Institute of Nursing' at Guy's Hospital. This trained women to nurse under Quaker influence. Later, Florence Nightingale, after her epic work in the Crimea, founded the Nightingale Training School at St. Thomas', which established three grades of nurses:

1. Sisters: in charge of a ward and carried out the orders of doctors, working also with probationer nurses.
2. Night superintendents: in charge of the night staff and deputized for matron.
3. Matron: responsible for employing and training nurses and for housekeeping and administration.

Other influences on nursing as it is today include the Poor Law Nursing Service (White, 1978), the Asylums (Carpenter, 1980), and, in the community, the Ladies Sanitory Reform Association in Manchester and Salford 1862 (Owen, 1977). This latter Association formed the origins of district nurses and health visitors.

From 1887 until the First World War, nurses struggled to obtain registration. The year 1916 saw the foundation of the College of Nursing and registration was finally obtained in 1919 by the Nurses' Registration Act. The College of Nursing was granted a royal charter in 1929. It is now the Royal College of

Nursing with headquarters in Cavendish Square, London and branches throughout England and Wales. A Scottish Board in Edinburgh and a Northern Ireland Committee in Belfast are local headquarters for the Scottish and Northern Ireland branches. In 1962 one united organization arose – the Royal College of Nursing and National Council of Nurses of the United Kingdom. This represents British nursing internationally.

Those training to become nurses must follow a course which lasts 3 years. This leads to the general nursing qualification, known as 'Registered General Nurse' (RGN). It provides a basis for later specialization and promotion. Some students choose to follow a different course – namely either mental nursing or mental handicap nursing courses. Successful completion of the respective three year courses leads to the qualification of 'Registered Mental Nurse' (RMN) and 'Registered Nurse for the Mentally Handicapped' (RNMH). A new system of nurse education, called Project 2000, is also underway in many parts of the UK. Nurses are regarded as 'registered practitioners' who start their training with an 18-month common foundation programme. This is followed by an 18-month 'branch programme' leading to registration on the general, paediatric, mental health or mental handicap parts of the Register. During training, students are educated to act as health promoters as well as caring for the sick. They are prepared for work in the community as well as in hospitals.

As well as Registered General Nurses, there are in the UK Enrolled Nurses and Nursing Auxiliaries. Enrolled nurses are less qualified than RGNs and Nursing Auxiliaries need no special qualifications at all. Project 2000 aims to convert all Enrolled Nurses into RGNs via a package of training. Similarly, Nursing Auxiliaries will cease to exist in favour of Health Care Assistants who will undertake a specific training programme.

In the US, nurse training results in a diploma, associate or baccalaureate degree. For nursing certain neurological conditions, some may specialize (after their initial training) in rehabilitation, perhaps with a masters degree or even a doctorate (Dittmar, 1989).

Community nursing

Community nursing developed through the voluntary organizations of the nineteenth century. Whereas hospital nurses followed doctors' orders regarding patient care, community nurses
worked more independently under the auspices of voluntary
organizations. In fact, the history of district nursing is closely
linked with William Rathbone in Liverpool and others such as
the Ranyard Nurses.

The Queen's Institute of District Nursing was founded with
money given to Queen Victoria in her Golden and Diamond
Jubilee. It accepted for training nurses who had completed the
basic training for registration or enrolment. In the late 1940s,
local health authorities became responsible for organizing the
home nursing services. Today the district nurse needs to obtain
a District Nursing Certificate in addition to her RGN training.
There are also District Enrolled Nurses.

The present community nursing service is organized so that
each nurse is responsible for a number of patients. This is
frequently based upon a particular family doctor's list. The district nurse assesses the patient, identifies priorities, constructs
and evaluates the care plan and uses the service of district
enrolled nurses and support workers to help her. She does not
stay with the patient but judges how often professional help is
needed. Thus she shares the delivery of care with relatives,
friends or other informal carers – all of whom she teaches and
supports. Often she works within a primary health care team
(see Chapter 8).

Occupational therapy

Occupational therapy covers any work or recreation and aims
to facilitate recovery from disease or injury (Levitt and Wall,
1992). Occupational therapists are concerned with physical,
neurological and psychiatric conditions. By selecting specific
activities and/or adapting the environment, they help people to
reach their maximum level of function in all aspects of daily
life. Their work, like nursing, is holistic. It encourages personal
well-being and meaningful relationships as well as physical
independence. It is a fairly recent discipline compared to others
in the medical and social fields. Nevertheless its concern with

the healing properties of work, exercise and play were recognized and used thousands of years ago (Mellis, 1990). Hopkins (1988) states that it is intimately related to humane treatment and began around the last quarter of the eighteenth century. During the French Revolution Phillippe Pinel introduced work treatment in the Bicetre Asylum for the Insane near Paris.

The term 'occupational therapy' originated in 1914 with George Barton, a founder member of the society that became the American Occupational Therapy Association. Under that name occupational therapy was first introduced into Britain in 1919 by Dr Henderson at the Glasgow Royal Mental Hospital, Gartnavel. Later on, it was used in the treatment of physical as well as mental conditions. In 1890, for example, Dr Philip of Edinburgh questioned the value of continued rest in the treatment of tuberculosis and advocated, instead, carefully prescribed exercise and activities. Occupational therapy advanced further during the First World War with Canada setting up a programme of occupational therapy. In Britain, Sir Robert Jones, an eminent surgeon, persuaded the War Office to set up orthopaedic centres. The success of his centre at Shepherd's Bush and the establishment of training schools at Bristol and Edinburgh in the 1930s encouraged the Ministry of health to set up rehabilitation workshops during the Second World War (Mellis, 1990).

The first professional association to be founded, in 1917, was the United States' national Soceity for the Promotion of Occupational Therapy. In 1923 this became the American Occupational Therapy Association which still exists today. In the UK, the Scottish Association of Occupational Therapists, formed in 1932, and the Association of Occupational Therapists, formed in England in 1936, united as the British Association of Occupational Therapists in 1974. This became an independent trade union in 1978 and the College of Occupational Therapists was formed to cater for the professional and educational aspects of the association's work. Nowadays training for occupational therapy lasts 3 years but there are plans to introduce degree courses in various parts of the country. Individuals may work in hospitals for the NHS or in the community for local authority social services. This community role developed partly as a result of the Chronically Sick and Disabled Persons Act, 1970, wherein local authorities were obliged to provide services for people registered as chronically sick or disabled (Mellis, 1990).

In the US, the start of occupational therapy can be traced to 1752 when the Pennsylvania Hospital was established. Benjamin Franklin, who was involved in this, suggested that inmates were provided with light manual labour (spinning and carding wool and flax). Nowadays, American occupational therapists qualify with a baccalaureate degree in occupational therapy, certified by the American Occupational Therapy Association (Dittmar, 1989).

Physiotherapy

Throughout history various physiotherapy techniques have been used in many countries – China, Egypt and Greece to name a few. Massage and rubbing are often mentioned. The term 'physiotherapy', however, was first used on 15 July 1905 in a letter in the *British Medical Journal* (Walton, 1990). Nowadays physiotherapy is considered to be the use of physical means to prevent and treat injury or disease and to assist rehabilitation (Levitt and Wall, 1992). The Chartered Society of Physiotherapy is the only recognized examining and professionial body for physiotherapists within the UK. It was founded in 1894 by four nurses fully trained in 'massage' and 'medical rubbing' who were concerned that their profession was falling into disrepute. There was at that time a craze for massage treatment, with newspapers publishing highly coloured stories about houses of ill fame. These masqueraded as nursing homes and lured young nurses into their precincts on the pretext of giving 'massage' to 'patients.' Even the British Medical Association published a warning against the use of massage in view of the number of unscrupulous and untrained people using it.

The four nurses were Lucy Robinson, Rosaline Paget, Elizabeth Manley and Margaret Palmer. They began to seek support amongst their colleagues for a Society which would restore 'massage' as an honourable profession. Hence in 1895, the 'Society of Trained Masseuses' was established. The first official examinations were held in February of that year. The Society became widely known in the medical world and in 1896 had selected medical doctors as its patrons. In 1900 it became the Incorporated Society of Trained Masseuses, acquiring the legal and public status of a professional organization.

In 1920 the Society merged with the rival Institute of Massage and Remedial Gynmastics and was granted a Royal Charter, becoming the Chartered Society of Massage and Medical Gymnastics. By then, membership was 5000 and the Society's patron was Her Majesty the Queen.

The current name, the Chartered Society of Physiotherapy (CSP) developed in 1942. This registered qualified practitioners, conducted exams and approved training schools. With the founding of the National Health Service in 1948, the CSP's training and examinations were approved as qualifications for employment in the NHS. The Chartered Society is the second oldest organization of physiotherapists in the world, the first being the Dutch. In November 1985, it merged with the Society of Remedial Gymnastics and Recreational Therapy. Physiotherapists may work either in hospitals or in the community. Training courses last 3 or 4 years.

In the US, physiotherapists are known as physical therapists. They qualify with a baccalaureate degree in physical therapy. Some continue to do a master's degree (1 – 2 years long), accredited by the American Physical Therapy Association (Dittmar, 1989).

Speech and language therapy

Speech and language therapy has existed as a profession only for a few decades. Its purpose is to identify and treat disorders of communication (Munro, 1990) and swallowing. Hitherto, disorders of speech were treated mainly by doctors, particularly stammering and deafness. However speech therapy advanced in the early twentieth century when the First World War produced numbers of head injured patients with speech disorders. In Britain the first speech clinic began at St Bartholomews' Hospital in 1911, followed by another at St Thomas' Hospital. Their directors were teachers of voice and speech and drama. Further hospital departments and local authority clinics were set up to offer treatment for a range of disorders. Speech and language therapists now identify, assess, and treat communication disorders in both children and adults. There has been debate for some time about whether the profession belongs to medicine or the field of education. This had led to argument and litigation.

Munro (1990) outlines the history of the profession. In the

UK two associations were founded. The first developed in 1934 from the remedial section of the Association of Teachers of Speech and Drama and was called the Association of Speech Therapists. The other, the British Society of Speech Therapists, was founded in 1935. They amalgamated in 1945 under the title of the College of Speech Therapists, which is the professional association for speech therapists today. The title of speech therapist was recently changed to speech and language therapists following a vote by members of the College (now known as the College of Speech and Language Therapists).

Speech and language therapists work mainly in the NHS, although some work in special schools or organizations or in private practice. Those in the NHS may be in hospital and/or community clinics, health centres and so on. Training involves a 4-year degree course. In the US, speech and language therapists are known as speech and language pathologists. They are certified by the American Speech and Hearing Association after completing a national examination in speech and language pathology and audiology. They must have a baccalaureate degree to practise but most specialize at master's or doctoral level.

Paramedical assistants or helpers

In the UK, many paramedical hospital departments employ unqualified staff. There are physiotherapy helpers, occupational therapy helpers or assistants, and, more rarely, speech and language therapy assistants. These individuals do not need to have any specialized knowledge to begin with. They are usually trained on the job, supervised by (and picking up various skills from) their senior paramedical professional colleagues. They are not usually involved in the assessment of patients but may be asked to carry out specified treatment programmes as well as various administrative duties.

The career structure for occupational therapy helpers is limited but exists from Helper through three grades to Technical Instructor I. Furthermore, occupational therapy helpers in the UK may qualify later as occupational therapists via a specific form of in-service training (providing certain conditions are fulfilled). Career structures for helpers and assistants in physiotherapy and speech and language therapy are less clear.

From 1990 onwards, however the three professional bodies for physiotherapy, occupational therapy and speech and language therapy have looked to the National Council for Vocational Qualifications (NCVQ) (National Council for Vocational Qualifications, 1989) to guide training, qualifications and competency standards for their support staff. Established in 1986, the NCVQ followed a government review of educational training. Its framework determines four levels of work activity that can be assessed. It relates these to National Vocational Qualifications (NVQs) and the paramedical professions continue to consult the framework of the NCVQ. In the US the American Occupational Therapy Association both sets the standards for and approves the training of occupational therapy assistants.

Clinical psychology

Psychology is the scientific study of behaviour and experience and clinical psychology is the application of this in the field of health care. The roots of modern psychology can be traced to the fourth and fifth centuries B.C. with the writings of the Greek philosophers Plato and Aristotle. However modern scientific psychology began around the middle of the nineteenth century. During that time, Wilheim Wundt, a German professor in Leipzig, and William James, an American professor in Cambridge, opened up laboratories of psychology. They began to train students in the science of human behaviour. Psychologists may follow one or many perspectives – behavioural, cognitive, psychoanalytic, phenomenological and biological. Each developed over time and offer different explanations of why individuals act as they do. Further discussion is available in Atkinson *et al.* (1990).

Clinical psychologists are involved in the assessment, treatment and management of emotional and behavioural problems. Cognitive disorders, for example memory deficits, can make up a large part of their caseload. They usually work directly with patients, either individually or in families or groups. They assess needs and provide therapies and help based on psychological theories and research. In the UK, they undertake a lengthy period of training and work before they are able to practise.

It takes at least 6 years to qualify as a chartered clinical psychologist. This involves first an honours degree in which psychology is the main subject followed by a professional training. This has both practical and academic components and leads either to a postgraduate degree or to the Society's Diploma in Clinical Psychology. Most clinical psychologists gain several years experience working in a relevant field before beginning their postgraduate clinical psychology training. The professional body for psychologists is The British Psychological Society and the Division of Clinical Psychology is one section of this. The Society was founded in 1901. It exists to promote the study of psychology and its applications and to maintain high standards of professional education and conduct.

In the US, a career in clinical psychology involves firstly a degree in psychology followed by a 5-year doctorate.

Social work

The development of social work in the UK has been distinctly haphazard. It emerged in different places as the need arose and was given different names. Barber and Kratz (1980) provide a summary of its history. The Probation Service, they say, was an early form of social work. This developed when church-affiliated court missionaries pleaded with magistrates to be allowed to reclaim drunkards rather than leave them to imprisonment or fine. In hospitals, 'almoners' were appointed. The word 'almoner' originally meant an official distributor of alms. Initially these people ensured that those who could afford to pay did not receive free treatment which, particularly in the teaching hospitals, was reserved for the poor. Gradually the almoner became more and more involved with complex social problems related to the patient's illness and his family. Thus she became known as a medical social worker and gradually started working with general practitioners and in local authority welfare departments as well as in hospitals. The first almoner to be appointed in the role of medical social worker was Mary Stewart. In 1895 she was allocated a dingy corner of the outpatients department of the London Royal Free Hospital. Over time almoners were appointed to most other general hospitals.

Another important influence on the development of social work as a profession was the Charity Organisation Society. This was established at the turn of the century to help those with little money who lived in poor housing conditions. The movement developed into the Family Welfare Association. The University Settlement movement also inspired the development of social work. Beginning with Toynbee Hall in the East End of London in 1884, this aimed to persuade university members to live and work in poor areas. Here they studied social conditions, conducted classes and tried to introduce certain reforms.

Hospital almoners, together with other groups such as psychiatric social workers, those concerned with residential and, in Scotland, probation officers, all amalgamated when social work departments were set up after the Second World War. These departments were organized on an area basis quite separate from medicine. This established a distinct profession which tried to distance itself from the image of the 'handmaidens of doctors' (Barber and Kratz, 1980). Thus social work gradually evolved in response to the problems of deprivation in an urban industrialized society. The social worker is responsible for helping patients and their families to deal with financial and emotional problems. She may also be able to give assistance with other practical issues, for example arranging of help for dependants (Garner, 1990).

There are two basic qualifications for the job of social worker – the Certificate of Qualification in Social Work (CQSW), a college-based course, and the Certificate in Social Service (CSS), a work-based route to social work. In addition a single qualifying award in social work to replace both these has been introduced. The Diploma in Social Work (DipSW) is being phased in and involves 2 years' training.

Dietetics

Dietetics is the science of diet and nutrition as applied to the feeding of groups and individuals in health and disease (Hyland and Hyland, 1990). The dietician's principal job is to tailor diet to the special needs of the patient, although education about diet is also an important feature. The first training schools for dieticians were established in the US in the 1920s. Their students were trained nurses. In Britain, the first dietetic department developed in Edinburgh in 1924, followed by the London Hospital in 1925. These early dieticians were nursing sisters, although the first graduate dieticians were recruited in 1928. In

1933 a special training course for dieticians was started at the King's College of Household and Social Science. At this time, the work mostly involved weighing and preparing foods. The British Dietetic Association was founded in 1936 and since then the dietician's work has expanded greatly. Dieticians work in the National Health Service in hospitals. The community dietician works with members of the Health Education Service, groups of the local population, the social services and the education services.

Training involves either a course for a degree in nutrition (with state registration in dietetics) or a degree in dietetics, both lasting 4 years. A 2-year postgraduate diploma course is also available.

PRESSURES WHICH RESTRICT TEAMWORK

On the team itself

Several factors may combine to prevent the smooth running of a team. The different attitudes of the various members are crucial because they will influence how the team works; for example the loner who prefers not to involve herself in the activities of others or who is defensive and territorial about her work, will limit her own and the team's potential. Conversely, 'compatible, "non-territorial" personalities' (Nieuwenhuis, 1990, p. 7) will be more prepared to use each other's expertise constructively, thus increasing their own knowledge and contributing to the team's overall success.

Edwards and Hanley (1989) list those features which limit interdisciplinary contact between occupational therapists and speech and language pathologists. This list is applicable to ALL members of the team and includes:

- severe staff shortage and staff changeover;
- financial constraints;
- physical barriers, such as the distance between departments and the various settings where they are located;
- the different philosophies of the member professions;
- conflict about the way cases should be handled;
- the opposition of administration and bureaucracy.

Smyth (1990) gives similar reasons which include matters of tradition, training and communication.

Another influence on the success of teamwork concerns the life experiences of the team members themselves – particularly with regard to health care. Some individuals may have been in hospital before or relied upon the community services. Therefore they may be in a better position to understand what it is like to be a patient. They may have first-hand experience of the devastating effects of disjointed team care. Hopefully this will assist their own efforts to provide a united team for the patient.

The following sections describe some of the pressures faced by various individuals. They are based on clinical experience and contact with fellow professionals. Frequently pressures like these conspire to make teamwork particularly difficult.

Pressures on the patient

The patient is a vital member of the team. He is the catalyst on which the others depend. Without him, the activities, status and careers of most of the professionals would cease to exist. Yet although several texts recognize his important role (Goodwill and Chamberlain, 1988; Fussey and Giles, 1988), he is often mentioned last, almost as an afterthought (Ashworth and Saunders, 1985; Wade *et al.*, 1985; Kaplan and Cerullo, 1986).

He faces many difficulties both in the hospital and in the community. His physical and mental state may prevent him from assuming responsibility for the decisions made on his behalf. Most probably, he will rely on the expertise of the professionals because he has neither the training nor the knowledge to make an informed choice. He may feel frightened and dependent. Others may encourage him, unconsciously, to assume and maintain the sick role. Accordingly he may become unmotivated to handle his own affairs (Granger and Gresham, 1984).

On the family

The family of the neurologically damaged patient is often in an uneveniable position (see Chapter 2 for comments raised by relatives themselves). They may have to provide physical care at home and may find this both physically and mentally exhausting. Emotional stress and disturbed family relationships may create further pressure, particularly if the patient suffers from behavioural and personality changes (Lezak, 1978; Livingston, 1986b). Families of patients with disabilities, however, should be included in the treatment process. A family can influence the outcome of rehabilitation (Granger and Gresham, 1984).

On the consultant

The consultant, who is accountable to the Regional Health Authority, has spent many years training and working to reach his current position. He has accumulated a vast amount of knowledge within a certain field and he is well aware of this. He is enveloped in a hospital hierarchy where patients, relatives and staff may perceive him to be the most important person involved in the patient's care. He alone holds overall clinical responsibility for the patient.

If he is over about 55 years of age, he is unlikely to have dealt significantly with the paramedical professions to any degree in his younger days. Therefore he may be unfamiliar with their self-acclaimed professional autonomy. Indeed he may resent the status which they assume when dealing with HIS patients on the ward. Furthermore the consultant faces several pressures in his job. These are described below.

1. Bureaucratic: in the UK, hospitals fight to survive in the face of government pressure to keep down their expenses. The consultant may be forced to justify the cost of treating his patient group. He may have to reduce his caseload as his bed allocation declines in competition with other specialities. Nursing staff on his ward may disappear preventing him from routinely admitting patients – as he has done in the past without question.
2. Time: he may be responsible for patients in other hospitals as well as having a community, a domiciliary and a private clinical commitment. He may even have a teaching commitment as well as trying to build up some research of his own.

On junior doctors

House officers and senior house officers in hospitals in the UK face their own pressures. As junior medical staff they work long hours performing vital but repetitive tasks such as clerking in patients and making provisional diagnoses, taking bloods, analysing test results, acting upon these appropriately, running outpatient clinics and various other duties. They must be ready to react to any medical emergency on the ward. They must be familiar with the status of all their patients and be able to summarize these for the consultant's ward round.

They may encounter death and terminal illness daily and have to deal with grieving and shocked relatives. This inevitably takes its emotional toll. The junior doctor may feel drained and exhausted both physically and emotionally. This will affect not only his performance at work (the demands of other staff become intolerable when he is tired) but also his ability to relax and enjoy himself after work. He may simply end up sleeping in order to recharge his batteries for his next shift. He may resent the effect that this, and his irregular hours, have upon his already limited social life. Other staff may appear to have an easier workload and more free time.

Furthermore, the junior medic may have had little or no contact with other paramedical staff. Even very recently in many UK medical schools, the only training he received about their roles throughout his long course, was an optional hour – on a day usually dedicated to sports activities. He may be unaware of both what they do and what they can offer the patient and his family. Accordingly he may assume that they are unimportant and that HE has more to contribute to patient care. He may even model himself on the consultant for whom he works and resent the status which paramedical staff claim as their due.

On the registrar/senior registrar

The registrar or senior registrar works under similar pressure. He may be about to move on in his career. Accordingly he will want a favourable reference from the consultant for whom he works. Previous posts may be unimportant at this stage – he is only as good as his last job. Prviately, he may support nursing and paramedical staff. However he may be unable to express this openly for, by opposing the views of his consultant, he may jeopardize his career prospects.

On the GP

The GP works from his own practice which he owns in partnership with his GP colleagues. He is accountable only to the Family Practitioner Committee. He has no obligations to other medical or paramedical staff. Community physiotherapists, psychiatric nurses, occupational therapists, and speech and language therapists may visit his premises or run community clinics particularly if he works at a health centre. However, he may have little contact with any of them. His experience of working with others may be limited to contact with his own practice nurse and the community district nurses.

He may have had limited contact with paramedical staff throughout his training and none since starting work as a GP. Thus he may be unaware of what they can offer the patient and little spare time to find out, relying merely on his previous knowledge and assumptions. He may not refer cases. Where he DOES refer, his only subsequent contact may be through reading their reports. He may disagree with the content of these, in particular with recommendations for terminating treatment and/or placing a patient on review. However his heavy caseload may limit the time he has to follow this up by contacting the therapists involved.

His contact with the local hospital may be restricted to occasional referrals to consultants. He may be happy to hand over specialist care to the hospital consultant and concentrate on dealing with his own caseload and pressures.

On nursing staff

The nurse has her own pressures to contend with. Traditionally she is seen as the 'doctor's handmaiden' and must carry out the instructions of medical staff. A multitude of tasks compete for her attention, including the essential jobs of bathing, feeding, and toileting. Senior ward staff also deal with drug rounds, ward rounds, admissions and discharges and the demands of patients and their relatives (and other staff involved with the patients on the ward). Ward sisters must also contend with the pressures from their own professional hierarchy who may enforce disruptive (and therefore unwelcome) staffing and policy changes. Successfully communicating information to all the interested parties is at the hub of this kind of job.

Like the doctor, the nurse is confronted frequently with terminal illness and death. It is HER job to dress the dead body (perform 'last offices') and deal with the relatives. She must present a professional but sympathetic stance although she may be tired and emotionally fraught. She may be working at full stretch due to a shortage of staff and may have little time left to respond to the demands of her paramedical colleagues. These demands may breed resentment if they come from someone who is rarely seen on the ward.

Consider the following scenario. An early morning sputum specimen may be crucial to ascertain whether the patient has developed a chest infection or even pneumonia. The nurse may have to obtain this (as well as carrying out her other duties) because the physiotherapist has not yet started work at this early hour. The nurse may resent this extra burden. She may be unaware that the other professions may have responsibilities elsewhere. The speech and language therapist, for example, may have to cover other hospital wards and do domiciliary home visits as well.

Ignorance about each others' pressures can breed resentment and irritation between the different parties. The nurse is particularly vulnerable because she has greater contact with the patient than any other staff member. With the family, she is the vital helper – indeed the therapist can see the patient for only 3–5% of her waking time each week (Wade *et al.*, 1984). This fact, on top of all the other pressures outlined above, may colour the nurse's opinion about the work of her team colleagues. She may perceive their input as infrequent and inadequate and therefore worthless. The paramedical staff, on the other hand, may feel that the nurse should at least be trying to carry out some of their recommendations when they themselves are unavailable.

Thomas (1988) describes the situation where members of one profession undertake an activity which is not usually their own job – because a member of the appropiate profession is not available. She notes that this problem has never really been discussed. Smyth (1990) suggests that there is no satisfactory solution, she lists problems which can intervene, for example staffing pressure, emergencies and unexpected visitors. It is always the nursing profession, however, which provides continuity of care at least in hospital. The importance of the nurse as a member of the rehabilitation team is well documented. Indeed Henderson *et al.* (1990) argue for a postbasic course in rehabilitation. This would allow the nurse to enhance the activities of the ward team consistently throughout the day and at weekends.

On the hospital-based physiotherapist

Senior physiotherapists and occupational therapists may work in one ward and in one speciality in the hospital. Their junior colleagues may rotate around the hospital and in different locations every 4 months or so. Thus junior members may only build up a transitory relationship with the nursing staff on their ward – and this can take several weeks to develop. This practice disrupts the harmony of working with the same person and learning how to get on with them. Thus it interferes with teamwork.

Various other pressures impinge upon the paramedic. Frequently staff of all three professions are asked to take on again for treatment somebody whom they had already discharged. Their reasons for discharge may have been varied, for example evidence of a plateauing of recovery, illness preventing the patient from gaining any benefit from therapy and so on. Other staffs' misconceptions of what can be achieved in therapy may cause stress and conflict. In some cases, moreover, the referring doctor may simply have used the referral as a way of getting the family off his back. However this does not help the therapist who may know from the outset that there is nothing more she can offer the patient at this stage, save reassessment (as requested) and further review appointments.

Positioning and handling of patients has already been mentioned as a source of conflict between physiotherapists and nursing staff (see Chapter 1). The problem here stems partly from the different training of the professions involved. The physiotherapist may follow the Bobath method, which is a well-established neurophysiological approach to treatment (see Chapter 6). Its two main principles are (i) inhibition of unwanted muscle patterns (i.e. the primitive patterns of flexion in the upper limb and extension in the lower limb), and (ii) facilitation of the automatic reactions such as righting, equilibrium and protective extension (Thompson and Morgan, 1990). Correct positioning and posture is vital to ensure that the central nervous system receives feedback from normal movement. The nurse, however, may be unaware of the Bobath concept. This lack of understanding will create friction between the two professions.

On the occupational therapist

The occupational therapist is concerned with looking at the patient's functional skills, for example his ability to dress himself, feed himself, go to the toilet and so on. Her activities may conflict with those of the physiotherapist. Consider, for example, two opposing views about the use of a wheelchair. The occupational therapist, concentrating on making the patient as functionally independent as possible, may offer the patient a wheelchair, encouraging him to propel himself with his unaffected arm. The physiotherapist, on the other hand, may prefer him not to use that arm at all. She may feel that any action with it simply increases the tone in the affected side.

Similarly conflicts may arise between the occupational therapist and the nursing staff. The occupational therapist may advocate a certain regime which will help the patient to dress himself. The nurse, pushed for time at the weekend and on those days when the therapist is unavailable, may choose to dress the patient herself and get on with the next job she has to do.

On the speech and language therapist

The speech and language therapist has pressures too. She may be responsible for the whole hospital and also for community work. Her sessions in the hospital may be irregular and a small proportion of her total caseload. She may be struggling to manage her inpatient numbers. She may never get to know the ward staff who may resent the irregularity and scarcity of her visits, without knowing the reason behind them. They may be reluctant to offer her assistance in, for example, lifting patients up the bed and positioning them appropriately. Indeed she may feel intimidated by their unfriendliness and be reluctant to ask for help.

She may never meet the consultant and have fleeting contact with the medical staff. She may be forced to write her reports in the medical notes without having the opportunity to discuss face-to-face with the other staff the results of her assessment and the problems she and they have encountered. This may breed resentment. Others may perceive her as working totally in isolation rather than as a member of the team.

Her involvement in helping patients with dysphagia may be relatively recent. This is a developing field with new practices being developed. Advice and management strategies may change over just a few years. These may conflict with the practices of the nursing staff. Indeed the speech and language therapist's recommendations (for example the advice described earlier in this chapter) may seem ludicrous to the nurse – who has been feeding patients for years without the help of (and, in her eyes, the need for) any one else.

On paramedical helpers and assistants

Physiotherapy helpers, occupational therapy assistants and, more rarely, speech and language therapy assistants also work in hospitals in the UK. Their duties vary according to the departments for which they work. Generally, however, they have some degree of patient contact. They, too, should be considered essential members of the team. Frequently, however, their status on the ward is not high. Staff of other professions may consider them to be unimportant because they hold no professional qualification. This may mean that the assistant receives little or no information about anyone or anything. Advice from other professionals, nursing and medical decisions, and other relevant news may pass her by – possibly because no one ever thinks to tell her. She may simply have to rely on what she picks up by chance and on what her superior remembers to tell her.

This level of perceived low status may have a negative effect on the individual herself. She may doubt her own value because she is neither included in any decision making nor introduced to other senior professionals. She may develop low self-esteem due partly to this psychological isolation within her working environment. A further pressure may arise from shortages of qualified staff. These may force some assistants to work unsupervised for long periods.

On the social worker

The social worker may suffer, like the paramedical assistant or helper, because other professionals perceive her to be supplementary to essential team care. This may be due to several reasons. Firstly, she is not usually involved in medical or paramedical treatment. Doctors and therapists may concentrate on physical and cognitive progress (Lees, 1988), forgetting the importance of family dynamics at home after discharge or practical issues such as who is going to collect someone's pension.

Another pressure on the social worker is the size of her department and the way it is organized. Members of small departments are often responsible for vast sections of the hospital or the community. This limits the input they can give and whether they are able to cover for absent colleagues. Other staff may be ready to complain when there is no social worker present at, for example, a ward meeting or case conference. However they may fail to appreciate that shortage of staff makes attendance physically impossible. Some hospital social workers resent the role of 'bed-emptiers' which may be foisted upon them. They may be under enormous pressure to find the patient somewhere to go and may be unable, through circumstance, to meet these expectations.

On the clinical psychologist

The clinical psychologist may suffer because other staff do not appreciate the importance of her area of expertise. Medical and nursing staff, physiotherapists and others may concentrate on physical disorders at the expense of cognitive factors. This may happen because memory and concentration, to name just two, are less tangible and therefore less noticeable than, for example not being able to walk, talk or dress. Further potential pressures on the clinical psychologist relate to information management. Frequently she may be asked to see relatives. This may involve going over with them what they have been told by the doctor, rephrasing where necessary. For this, she must know what has been said and in what context. This may be difficult if she is not kept up to date with the latest developments. Situations like this may arise because other staff may not think to give her information, unaware, perhaps, that she is involved in the case at all. Limited appreciation by other staff may create tension and stress and have a negative influence on the psychologist's interaction with the team.

On the community paramedical professional

The community physiotherapist, occupational therapist and speech and language therapist may experience similar problems to those of their hospital colleagues. Contact with each other may be limited. Indeed, in some cases, members of two community professions may never even see each other – although their visits to the patient's house may simply be an hour apart. This has implications for the communication of information and hence for the success of team care. Wade (1987) illustrates the problem when he asks how, for example, does the part-time speech therapist communicate with the part-time district nurse?

A united source of record keeping would help to reduce this problem and will be discussed elsewhere (see Chapter 4). Most community professionals, however, simply have to struggle on without this, relying on the telephone to contact other people. Often the person they are trying to reach is unavailable at the time they themselves have access to a phone. This means that communication is delayed and perhaps abandoned as other pressures mount up. Contact by letter takes longer and loses the personal touch of the telephone.

Other practical pressures confront the community professional. They may spend much of their time driving around on domicilary visits and trying to find adequate parking space. This may be both stressful and tiring. They may have little time to write up their patient's notes and they may have to transport and store much equipment in their cars.

Difficulties like these are voiced by others. Smyth (1990) stresses that multidisciplinary work is even more difficult for the community professional than the hospital-based professional because '. . . conscious thought must be given to arranging the necessary one-off joint-visits or case-conferences. Even getting to know the identity of the other professionals and carers who are working round a particular client can be difficult' (p. 131). Jones (1992) lists social, environmental and psychological difficulties for the community physiotherapist which apply readily to anyone doing a community job.

On the dietician

Pressures on dieticians usually stem from lack of awareness and, often sheer ignorance, about the full range of their activities. Much of their work involves educating patients about a diet, tailored to suit individual needs. However, this aspect may take place with the patient alone, unseen and, therefore, unacknowledged by other members of staff. Fellow professionals may simply use the dietician as a source of supply for meals and nasogastric or gastrostomy feeds.

Further stress may stem from complaints by relatives and staff about hospital food. A purée diet, for example, may 'look unappetizing', be considered too runny or contain unsuitable pieces of soft food. Similarly, food may be cold, tasteless or there may not be enough of it. However these and other such problems may stem from difficulties in the catering rather than the dietetic department. Such misunderstanding may lead to resentment and hostility.

A further problem voiced by dieticans is lack of available up-to-date information. A patient's medical notes, for example, may fail to record that a nasogastric tube is no longer *in situ*, the patient having removed it earlier in the day. Essential facts like these will influence directly the dietician's treatment plan and yet may not be passed on to her unless she happens to meet staff on the ward. This lack of communication can be expensive (nasogastric feeds are still provided from the dietician) and a waste of professional time.

CONCLUSION

This chapter has set out to share information between the disciplines who care for the adult with acquired neurological brain damage. It assumes that mutual awareness may promote greater understanding between the professionals involved. Thus the first part outlines the historical development of each profession. Subsequent sections describe the pressures which individuals may face in their daily work. Comments are based on clinical experience and discussion with colleagues from other disciplines.

4

Assessment

. . . each discipline thinks it understands exactly what all the other disciplines do.

Thomas 1988, p. 123.

Assessment is an activity common to all professionals involved in caring for the neurologically brain-damaged adult. It involves evaluation of both the patient's condition and relevant factors pertaining to it (for example physical features such as 'hearing', psychological ones such as 'mood', and social factors such as 'home circumstances'). Each profession, however, tends to concentrate on different parameters – depending upon its area of expertise. The clinical psychologist, for example, will concentrate on the assessment of cognition, where the speech and language pathologist will be interested in communication. The nurse, because she is involved in care of the whole patient, takes a holistic approach, assessing a wide range of factors, medical and social (see Chapter 3 for a summary of the areas of expertise of each profession).

Students spend much of their training learning about assessment and its interpretation. Indeed the ability to perform accurate assessment of a specific area in a particular way is an important feature distinguishing the different professions from one another. Formal assessments, which test specific areas, for example language or perception, allow systematic and objective evaluation of the patient's performance (Garner, 1990). Results are standardized on a specific population and can be quantified. Examples of these are the Rivermead Perceptual Assessment Battery (RPAB) (Whiting *et al.*, 1985), used primarily by occupational therapists and the Western Aphasia Battery (Kertesz, 1982), used by speech and language therapists.

Informal assessments, on the other hand, are subjective and offer more qualitative results. They are not standardized but describe, at a specific time, the unique performance of the individual who is being assessed. Many paramedical therapists have developed their own informal tests in the course of their work and use these as handy assessment tools in clinic. In addition much of their informal assessment and also the assessment performed by nursing staff may be based on observation. Indeed there is no other means of testing which is so potentially accurate in the right hands (Carr and Shepherd, 1980).

Obviously there are several areas of overlap between the tests used by the different professions. This chapter will describe a range of the assessment parameters of doctors, nurses, physiotherapists, occupational therapists, speech and language therapists, clinical psychologists, social workers and dieticians. Some of the individual tests themselves are mentioned. The latter sections will pinpoint areas of overlap, potential problems which arise, and ways of improving communication about assessment results.

THE DOCTOR'S ASSESSMENT

The house officer and/or senior house officer is involved in clerking admissions. For this, he has a set history and examination framework. This can vary slightly between different hospitals but it generally includes the following features:

1. Biographical details.
2. Route of referral, e.g. emergency, via clinic etc.
3. Presenting complaint. This is usually in brief and in the patient's own words.
4. History of presenting complaint.
5. Past medical history.
6. Family history.
7. Social history.
8. Systems review. This is a brief and fairly comprehensive interrogation which covers the cardiovascular system, respiratory system, gastrointestinal tract, urogenital system and the central nervous system.

From these parameters, the doctor reaches a provisional diagnosis of the patient's problem. Several investigations may be required to confirm this or to provide further information. Referral to other specialist departments may also be necessary.

NURSING ASSESSMENT

Until the early 1960s, many nurses supposed that professional nursing practice should rely upon instinct and empathy. However in 1963, Bonney and Rothberg were among the first to call for more systematic assessment of patients and their needs. They thought that the physical, psychological and behavioural aspects of an individual were particularly important (Aggleton and Chalmers, 1986). This way of thinking eventually resulted in 'The Nursing Process' (Yura and Walsh, 1967).

The nursing process provides the basis of nursing assessment in the UK today. It distinguishes a discrete number of stages in nursing care which include:

1. Assessment – of physiological, psychological and social aspects.
2. Planning – of short-term, intermediate, or long-term goals.
3. Intervention – to help patients achieve these goals.
4. Evaluation – of what the patient can do at a particular point compared with the goals previously set.

Thus, the nursing process is a cyclical one. Further nursing problems are identified throughout the patient's stay in hospital and evaluation of care implies the reassessment of the patient.

Generally nurses do not rely on standardized tests. There may be several reasons for this. Firstly such tests are often lengthy and unwieldy and therefore inappropriate for use in a busy ward or, where the district nurse is concerned, at the patient's home. Furthermore standardized tests tend to tackle specialist areas (for example cognition or language). Detailed analysis of individual areas like these is not the nurse's concern. She is more interested in getting an overall view of what the patient can and cannot do, taking account of any relevant social and psychological factors. This is because she is the only person in a position to provide continuity of care whilst the patient is in hospital (Thomas, 1988). A holistic rather than a specialist assessment is crucial.

Much of her assessment takes the form of observation (for example the patient's colour, nutritional state, skin condition and so on), recording of factual information (for example whether the patient is continent) and informal questioning. Detailed assessment is necessary if the patient is seriously ill or unconscious – in which case it is also necessary to collect information from relatives or a friend. For all patients, temperature, pulse, respiration and blood pressure levels are recorded and charted on admission as well as the result of urinalysis. Whilst 'clerking in' a patient, the nurse records her assessment results on a nursing Kardex form. In this way she is able to construct a patient profile on which to base a nursing care plan. This plan is a hierarchical method of controlling the order in which a sequence of operations is performed. It is a written record of identified nursing problems and the nursing actions to be taken to meet the patient's needs. The areas covered by the nurse in her initial assessment include:

1. biographical details;
2. health information, including present diagnosis (if known), symptoms, past health problems, previous admissions to hospitals, allergies and so on;
3. the patient's perception of the reason for admission, his view of hospital admission, whether there is anything he is worried about or particularly fears;
4. the patient's description of the usual pattern of daily living habits such as sleep, diet, activity, bowel habits and so on.

There are also some scoring tests which the nurse may use. An example is The Norton Scale (Norton *et al.*, 1962). This is a simple and reliable way of evaluating a patient's general condition and his liability to develop pressure sores. The patient is assessed on each of five variables, namely, physical condition, mental condition, activity, mobility and incontinence. He obtains a score from one to four on each of these. Scores are then added. The lower the patient's total score, the greater the risk that he will develop a sore: any patient with a score lower than 14 is at risk, while a score lower than 12 indicates a particularly worrying level of risk. The scoring system can be used to determine how often pressure areas should be attended to (Clarke, 1991).

PHYSIOTHERAPY ASSESSMENT

Parry (1980) outlines three areas of the physiotherapist's assessment:

1. Subjective examination

This involves listening to the patient. Crucial factors are his description of his illness and disability, how it has progressed, how it has interfered with his lifestyle and what previous conditions might have precipitated or influenced it. Other relevant information includes the use of drugs and their effects, previous medical history and social factors.

2. Objective examination

This involves collecting all relevant information through observing, palpating and testing. General areas which should be covered include behaviour and orientation, muscle tone, posture, quality of movement, involuntary movement, gait, functional ability, dexterity and communication. Local areas of assessment include skin condition, pain, muscle wasting, joint stability, contractures and deformities, and movement. Other tests and measurements look at motor responses (for example spinal reflexes, tonic reflexes, automatic postural adjustment, range of movement, muscle strength and electrical reactions.) Finally there should be at least some assessment of sensation, coordination, visual field defects, perception and cognition.

3. Interpretation

This is crucial because the accurate interpretation of any abnormalities of structure and function allows the planning of appropriate treatment. Parry (1980) suggests listing problems in order of priority, then establishing aims of treatment. This allows the therapist to consider, next, the means by which these aims can be met. Throughout treatment, reassessment is important because it may indicate that the treatment programme needs modification.

Physiotherapists use a wide range of assessments which are generally very detailed. Members of other professions may find them difficult to understand because they do not have the specialist knowledge required. Therefore they may need to spend a substantial amount of time trying to learn about them. As a basic assessment, Allen *et al.* (1988) advocate use of the Motricity Index (Demeurisse *et al.*, 1980) coupled with a modified measure of trunk control. The physiotherapist will obviously add her own in-depth assessments to these to obtain a detailed picture of the patient's skills.

OCCUPATIONAL THERAPY

The literature on occupational therapy categorizes, in different ways, the assessment areas of the profession. Spencer (1983), when discussing head injury, lists eleven parameters. These are given below: Areas of Assessment in Occupational Therapy:

- Communication;
- Behaviour;
- Social;
- Auditory;
- Visual;
- Sensory;
- Physical;
- Functional;
- Educational;
- Vocational;
- Driver evaluation.

Adapted from Spencer (1983).

Other authors emphasize different topics depending upon the neurological condition under discussion. Thompson and Morgan (1990) categorize the important areas in the assessment of stroke as:

1. personal activities of daily living – this includes eating and drinking, toileting, washing and dressing, grooming and bathing;
2. sensory function;
3. perception;
4. domestic activities of daily living.

Garner (1990) includes aspects of physical dysfunction (namely positioning, spasticity, ataxia, muscular weakness or paralysis, range of movement and other features.) She also lists psychosocial aspects (personality change, behaviour, effects on the family and cognitive impairment) which are crucial in acute head injury, the subject of her text.

Occupational therapists are concerned with activities of daily living (ADL) and there are a great many ADL indexes and scales. The idea of ADL is that it assesses the ability of the patient to care for himself physically (Allen *et al.*, 1988). It does not normally cover a patient's social independence, although some scales do include homework tasks.

The Barthel Index is probably the best known and has been used in stroke research. For succinct descriptions of the index, see Wade (1986) and Allen *et al.* (1988). Both favour its use for several reasons. It contains all the generally accepted ADL items, is the most widely used ADL index in stroke research, is a valid and probably reliable measure and forms a hierarchical scale (the same score usually implies the same abilities). Furthermore, they say, it is probably a useful tool in assessing other neurological diseases. Critics of the Barthel Index point to its insensitivity. A patient may well be able to stand upright but this may take great effort and time, features not reflected within the final score.

The Chessington OT Neurological Assessment Battery (COTNAB) (Tyerman *et al.*, 1986) is one of the standardized tests used by some occupational therapists. It consists of 12 separate tests within the categories of (i) visual perception (ii) constructional ability (iii) sensory-motor ability and (iv) ability to follow instructions. For further discussion of this test see Thompson and Morgan (1990) who also list tests for identifying disability in stroke patients. Another standardized test is the Rivermead Perceptual Assessment Battery (RPAB) (Whiting *et al.*, 1985).

SPEECH AND LANGUAGE THERAPY ASSESSMENT

Assessment of communication and swallowing ability are the two main concerns of the speech and language therapist. Several features are important in assessing these areas.

Assessment of communication encompasses the following:

1. Assessment of oral-motor function: relevant parameters include:
   (a) respiration;
   (b) laryngeal activity;
   (c) palate;
   (d) tongue;
   (e) lips;
   (f) intelligibility;
   (g) sensation;
   (h) reflex activity (i.e. the presence of a cough reflex).
2. Assessment of language: this involves consideration of:
   (a) auditory comprehension (i.e. understanding of the spoken word);
   (b) verbal expression or speech;
   (c) non-verbal communication (including use of gesture, facial expression and body movement);
   (d) reading;
   (e) writing;
   (f) environmental variables such as the communicative setting. This includes factors such as noise levels, lighting, the opportunity to speak to other people and so forth. These will all affect the success of communication;
   (g) alternative methods of communication, for example the use of a 'Lightwriter'. This is a small, portable communication aid with a keyboard on which the patient spells out messages. These are displayed simultaneously on two visual display screens, one facing the patient and the other facing the person who is 'listening'.

The assessment of swallowing ability will include all the parameters tested in (1) above. In addition, the speech and language therapist will need to consider the patient's mental state, the history of the problem, diet, posture, the swallow reflex (both spontaneous and in response to the introduction of liquid and foods of varying consistency), chest condition and other factors.

She will also look at various features of mental status as these, too, may affect communication or swallowing ability. Attention, visual and auditory acuity, mood, orientation and memory are important areas which should be observed.

There are a staggering variety of both formal and informal

assessments. Those used will depend upon the age and condition of the patient, the nature of the problem (is the patient dysphasic, dysarthric, demented or dysphagic?) and what information is sought. Standardized tests for aphasia include The Boston Diagnostic Aphasia Examination (Goodglass and Kaplan, 1972) and the Western Aphasia Battery (Kertesz, 1982) to name just two. There are also several informal tests available. One approach, called the 'cognitive neuropsychological assessment of aphasia' relies heavily on these and is based on complex theories of language processing.

Functional communication refers to the ability to communicate by using all available parameters. Assessments look at the way a patient can interpret situations and respond to them in a meaningful way. This includes not only speech but gesture, context, facial expression and so on. Several informal tests are available, for example the Edinburgh Functional Communication Profile (Wirz *et al.*, 1992). The assessment of dysarthria also tends to rely on more informal tests such as the Frenchay Dysarthria Assessment (Enderby, 1988) or the Dysarthria Profile (Robertson, 1982).

The bedside assessment of swallowing difficulties relies heavily on subjective, informal information gained as part of an overall clinical evaluation. In addition a more objective radiological investigation may be performed. This is known as a 'modified barium swallow with videofluoroscopy'. It is performed by qualified radiologists although the specialist speech and language therapist may assist. In fact several hospitals have established 'dysphagia clinics' where modified barium swallows with videofluoroscopy are carried out regularly on suitable patients to aid diagnosis and management of swallowing problems.

Further information about the speech and language therapist's assessment activities is available in Umphred (1985).

DIETETIC ASSESSMENT

Dieticians use their knowledge of nutrition, medicine and social science to devise appropriate eating patterns for people in hospital and in the community. Their assessment uses a number of methods. A diet history is obtained from the patient or carers and, if in hospital, the patient's eating and drinking is monitored by nursing staff when possible. The dietician also notes the patient's weight, records recent weight changes and calculates the body mass index. She uses medical and biochemical information to determine a therapeutic diet where necessary. Social circumstances are also considered, therefore a holistic approach is used.

SOCIAL WORK ASSESSMENT

The social worker can play a crucial role in the management of the adult with an acquired neurological disease. Often, social, emotional and psychological factors are those which create the greatest difficulties for the patient and his relatives both at home and in the hospital (see Chapter 2). Therapists and doctors, however, tend to perceive progress primarily in physical terms (Lees, 1988), probably because this is what they have been trained to assess and treat. It is part of the emphasis, and understandably so, of their professional expertise.

The social worker (and the clinical psychologist), on the other hand, are those most equipped to assess and deal with psychosocial difficulties. Indeed, with regard to assessment, the social worker, of all the professions, is the person who probably relies most on informal intervention. This includes assessment of the situation and the crucial subjective factors (for example relations between patient and spouse, financial security) which dictate whether the patient may live satisfactorily at home or not.

Thus the social worker's assessment may exist in the form of informal notes and observations. Talking, listening and observing are crucial activities in this type of work and should not be frowned upon just because they are subjective and 'unscientific' in form. Indeed they often provide the key to successful rehabilitation or even whether patient and family can cope with terminal illness at home. Standardized testing, with its scientific rigour, may be unsuitable and irrelevant in situations like this.

Instead of formal assessments, such as those described in the sections above, the social worker relies on feelings, intuitions, and practical issues. Basic arrangements such as care for the patient's dog during hospitalization need to be tackled and by someone who knows what can be done. The social worker can assess what is important in the patient's life. These are important issues whose successful assessment and management can play a crucial part in the patient's well-being and thereby in his attitude to therapy.

In general, formal testing often requires lengthy interviews, time and form filling, both on the part of the patient and the assessor. The social worker, on the other hand, tends to base her assessment on her analysis of conversation and interviews with the patient and significant others in his immediate environment. Her observations are often made in the patient's home.

CLINICAL PSYCHOLOGICAL ASSESSMENT

The clinical psychologist has a vast array of formal and informal tests at her disposal. The choice of which one to use will depend upon the age and medical diagnosis of the patient, and the topic which needs to be assessed (for example memory, anxiety, mental state).

If memory is the problem, objective assessments are generally of very little value and will not give the assessor information on how the patient performs. However, functional tests, such as the Rivermead Behavioural Memory Test (Wilson *et al.*, 1985) assess the patient's ability to remember names, routes, instructions, faces, stories and where things are put. They measure the problem in practical terms (Garner, 1990). Examples of other tests include the Kendrick Cognitive Tests for the Elderly (Kendrick, 1985) and the Beck Depression Inventory (Beck, 1988).

AREAS OF OVERLAP WITHIN ASSESSMENT

Obviously each profession has its own particular area of expertise (see Chapter 3). The above sections illustrate how different professional assessments concentrate on different areas; however, they also show overlap. Most professions include some basic information about social details, behaviour and communication (assessed in more detail by the social worker, clinical psychologist and speech and language therapist, respectively). Similarly, everyone relies on the medical information provided by the doctor.

Other areas overlap between the different professions to a lesser extent but are still assessed by more than one person. The nurse and the physiotherapist both cover some basic points of ADL, although the occupational therapist specializes in this area. Similarly, positioning is assessed in different ways and to different degrees by the physiotherapist and the occupational therapist. Yet the nurse and the speech and language therapist also cover this area. The nurse, for example, needs to know the best position for the patient if his skin is in danger of breaking down and the speech and language therapist is interested in the best possible posture for swallowing and feeding.

There are further areas of overlap. The assessment of perception is covered by both the occupational therapist and the clinical psychologist. Sensation is assessed by the occupational therapist, physiotherapist and the doctor. Spasticity is evaluated primarily by the physiotherapist and the occupational therapist, although the nurse and the doctor also look at this area more superficially. Finally the ability to eat and drink is also assessed by the nurse, the occupational therapist and the doctor, although the speech and language therapist looks at this area in much greater detail.

Obviously each profession evaluates these areas in different ways. The very fact that there is overlap, however, creates potential for acrimony amongst members of the team. One person may resent the fact that others, less qualified, have made a superficial assessment of her area of expertise. Written comments on communication, for example, may irritate the speech and language therapist particularly if they contradict her own views, based on her detailed assessment of this area. Subconsciously she may be defensive about her professional territory. Conflicting remarks about the patient's posture, recorded in the medical notes by the physiotherapist, occupational therapist, nurse and speech and language therapist (assessed by them in different ways) can lead to further bad feeling.

Many readers, justifiably, will argue that acrimony like this over assessment merely reflects a disunited team. This may well be so. Nevertheless written communication of assessment results is often the only point of regular contact between everyone involved in the patient's care. Part-timers may find this a particular problem because they may not work on the days of ward meetings, case conferences and so on. The lack of opportunity to meet and discuss assessment may inspire some people simply to ignore the results of others, especially where there are areas of overlap. Unfamiliarity with and ignorance of each other's assessment techniques may heighten this response.

The casualties are the patient and his family. Overlap like this has practical implications for them. Multiple assessment by different professionals of one parameter provides fertile ground for duplication and redundancy. Unless there is good communication between the team members, patient and family may end up answering repeatedly the same type of questions about the same topic.

Picture the patient who is assessed by the doctor in accident and emergency and who is admitted to hospital. He is then assessed in the same way by the house officer or senior house officer who 'clerks him in' on the ward. Next he faces a 'clerking in' by nursing staff. This assessment and examination may be slightly different from those he has just undergone – twice – but he may not perceive this to be the case in the circumstances. Furthermore he may wonder why he has to repeat himself and why the staff fail to tell each other the facts, which, he observed, were written down at the first assessment anyway.

He may then be referred for X-ray investigation, encountering thereby a specialist doctor who assesses him medically – for a third time. Later, physiotherapists and occupational therapists may pounce. By this time, he may have answered questions about, for example, his symptoms or his home background, five times. He has yet to meet the social worker and other members of the team. He may conclude, with justification, that his care is unnecessarily labour intensive. He may readily appreciate why everyone assesses their own speciality in depth; however, he may resent superficial assessment of the same topics by different people. He may have entered hospital perceiving it as one organization. Unfortunately, reporting something once to one worker in the system does not lead to everyone receiving the information. If it did, the organization would be much more streamlined and efficient.

IMPROVING COMMUNICATION IN ASSESSMENT

One way of getting round this is to try to improve communication in assessment. Doctors may not need to reassess the patient in exactly the same way so often. Perhaps they could relieve the burden on the patient by only reassessing those areas which are crucial, digesting first the information written previously by their medical colleagues.

Another step might be to reduce the plethora of obscure tests used by different professionals. Wade has been a staunch advocate of a basic uniform assessment package in the field of stroke. Limiting initial testing to specific tests and measures prevents redundancy such as that listed above. Furthermore it improves communication between professionals as they all get to learn exactly how another profession works. This can help to guarantee a unified approach, particularly where there are areas of overlap between the professions (Lynch and Grisogono, 1991).

Wade (1992), Allen *et al.* (1988) and Wade (1986) suggest a set battery of tests to improve stroke care. The exact nature and number of these varies with the individual authors but generally include the following:

1. The Barthel Index (Mahoney and Barthel, 1965) to describe the patient's ADL ability.
2. The Frenchay Aphasia Screening Test (Enderby *et al.*, 1987), to detect aphasia and describe its severity.
3. The Motricity Index (Demeurisse *et al.*, 1980) and Trunk Control Test (Sheikh *et al.*, 1980) to measure motor function.
4. The Hodkinson Mental Scale (Hodkinson, 1972) to detect and describe confusion.
5. The Rivermead Perceptual Assessment (Whiting *et al.*, 1985) to clarify perceptual problems when clinically indicated.
6. The Frenchay Activities Index to describe the extent of any return to former social activities.
7. The Rivermead Mobility Index (Collen *et al.*, 1991) to evaluate mobility. Measuring the time taken to walk 10 metres is also useful.
8. Star Cancellation (Halligan *et al.*, 1989) to assess for the presence of neglect.

Wade (1987) discusses again the thorny problem of assessment measures, focusing on the practice of paramedicals. He argues that the absence of any common language renders communication impossible, and he gives Oxfordshire as an example. Within this area at least ten different ADL forms are used and the variety of physiotherapy assessments is legion. Wade has some strong comments to make. The measures used are rarely tested for validity or reliability. Those published, he says, are often too long and complex for routine use, irrelevant to others and quite incommunicable. He concludes that while no uniform set of measures exists, no one profession will be able to understand, or be understood by, other professions, and each person will tend to ignore the work of others.

Allen *et al.* (1988) fuel the cry for a uniform battery of assessment in the field of stroke. They argue that the physician does not need to assess or describe the disability himself. He should insist, however, that other professionals do so using simple measures with which he is familiar.

Such comments may provoke strong reaction from therapists. They may resent being told what to do, and perceive this both as a threat to, and an invasion of, their professional autonomy. Furthermore they may believe that assessment, such as that proposed, is often inappropriate given the patient's condition. Another criticism is that it fails to measure the idiosyncratic qualitative differences in a patient's individual performance. These characteristics often have more significance for the patient and his recovery than objective figures gained during standardized testing. Indeed, more uniform assessment has been tried before, at least in the field of occupational therapy. Squires and Taylor (1988) describe an attempt by the British Association of Occupational Therapists to standardize ADL forms. Their efforts were unsuccessful. Occupational therapy departments preferred their own ADL forms which had been designed to reflect local needs.

Nevertheless, Allen *et al.* (1988) are not totally negative about the variety of paramedical assessment currently used. They DO admit that additional in depth testing may be useful in investigating the patient's problems further and in planning subsequent treatment. They merely argue that a common assessment base, which everybody understands, provides better communication. Improved communication is necessary for effective team work (see Chapters 1 and 3) and therefore Allen *et al*'s remarks, however controversial, deserve consideration.

Garner (1990), herself an occupational therapist, has further comments relevant to improving communication in assessment. She does not advocate a uniform battery of tests. However she does stress that all therapists should get to know each others' methods of assessment. This facilitates understanding of what the person actually does. One way of doing this, she says, is for two therapists, of different professions, to do an assessment together. One person can actually work with the patient and the other can record the responses. This type of assessment is particularly valuable because the two professionals will have different skills. Chapter 8 of this book provides practical examples of joint assessment like this.

RECORDING ASSESSMENT RESULTS

Recording assessment results presents further problems. All members of the team usually consult the medical notes and write reports in these when necessary. However most therapists keep separate notes in their own departments. Nurses, on the other hand, record information in a nursing Kardex system and/ or nursing care plan on the ward. Unfortunately individuals rarely peruse each others' records. Indeed they may have neither the opportunity nor the inclination. They may even question whether they are entitled to do so.

The number of professional records which are used can hamper the efficient communication of information. Sometimes a vital piece of information, often about the patient's social predicament, fails to reach the medical notes – usually the only source consulted by all team members. The nurse may learn, for example, that the patient's sibling is dangerously ill. She may make a note of this in the nursing Kardex. However the information, lying hidden in her professional records, may remain inaccessible to the clinical psychologist who has been asked to assess whether the patient is suffering from depression. He may only consult the medical records never considering the nurse's system at all.

Breakdown in the transfer of information will most likely occur UNLESS all news is always recorded in every set of professional notes relating to the patient. This is hardly practical. Indeed this practice may be compounded by territorial rights and behaviour and legal and ethical implications. The result is that, for example, the nurse may never look at the physiotherapist's assessment results. Similarly the clinical psychologist may never see the nursing care plan which may contain crucial up-to-date information on the patient 's current mental state. Information, of course, may be passed by word of mouth at ward rounds and case conferences. However this method of communication is unreliable if different people are available at different times. Their paths may not cross during the course of the week. Successful transfer of information may be haphazard and even depend upon everyone's off-duty rota.

Moreover, a lot of information will be duplicated. Each profession may end up copying relevant information from another source into their own notes. They may even triplicate their own comments in an attempt to reach all members of the team. They may write, for example, in the medical notes for the doctor, in the nursing Kardex for the nurse and in their own departmental notes. This procedure is labour intensive and redundant. One way of getting around the problem of communicating up-to-date information to everybody is to use one set of notes for all professions. Assessment results and ongoing progress notes could be recorded just once to avoid duplication and redundancy. Free access and the chance to add any relevant information might improve communication between professionals and hence enhance team care.

POMR AND 'SOAP' NOTES

'Problem orientated medical recording' (POMR) is one such system available. Described by Parry (1980), Winterton and Haldane (1988), and Ransome (1990), this was first introduced by Dr Lawrence Weed in 1969. It was originally developed as a total patient care medical record, with a structured written input from all disciplines. These related to a clearly defined list of an individual patient's problems. The system records information in a logical format. It consists of four main headings (although Smyth, 1990, adds a fifth one).

These are described below.

1. Database: a record of all relevant subjective and objective information, including the patient's personal details, his medical and social histories and results of objective examination.
2. Problems list: a comprehensive list of the patient's problems built up from information recorded in the database.

3. Initial plan: a programme of total care for the patient, planned by referring to the problem list.
4. Progress notes: these can be recorded as a flow chart or, more commonly as narrative notes. The narrative notes are written under four headings – subjective, objective, assessment and plan. They are sometimess called SOAP notes because of the anacronym formed by the initials of these four headings.
5. Discharge summary (added by Smyth, 1990).

Parry (1980), Winterton and Haldane (1988) and Smyth (1990) all provide further information about how the system works. Smyth outlines the benefits. It allows more orderly and comprehensive patient care. It prevents not only problems from being overlooked but also the duplication of therapeutic effort. She maintains, however, that it is rarely used in specialist units, let alone general hospitals. Expanding her remarks further, it is hard to envisage the use of this system in the community. One major problem would be where to store the notes themselves. Therapists and social workers frequently work in different locations from both each other and from GPs and nurses, who are also involved in the patient's care. Furthermore they might all need the notes on the same day, although at different times.

POMR does have other disadvantages. Cantrell (1988) points out that it concentrates on the negative side of the person – with what is wrong. He maintains that it should really include a list of all disabilities, practical outcomes of the condition (job impossible, inadequate finance and so on) rather than be restricted to medical comments. Furthermore it excludes family details which signify the context from which a person comes and the people who end up being the helpers in community life (see Chapter 2). Cantrell advocates, instead, the use of the Southampton Household Matrix System (Cantrell and Dawson, 1983). This records both positive and negative factors for the patient and the main helpers.

CONCLUSION

Assessment is a major issue in any discussion of teamwork. It is vital because it highlights what the patient can and cannot do – and therefore guides the team members as to how they can help. The sections above illustrate that although each profession concentrates on its own area of expertise, there is also overlap to varying degrees. This overlap can become a source of frustration for the patient and his family – particularly where channels of communication between professionals are poor.

There are some ways of alleviating the problem. Team members might choose to unite in the way proposed by Wade. They might decide to use a set number of well-known and established assessments as part of their initial testing routine. This might improve communication and understanding between team members. However, recording assessment results is also an issue which needs to be addressed. The use of separate professional notes can lead to duplication, redundancy and inadequate transfer of information. The team needs an efficient way of communicating assessment results. POMR is one system that is available, although this is neither widely used nor without its own faults.

5

Approaches, models and techniques

Chapter 3 has described the different histories of the professions. It illustrates how medicine, nursing, clinical psychology, the three paramedical professions, dietetics and social work have each developed their own identity over the years. During this time some have also developed their own models. Indeed the concept of a model is now thought to be an important issue in many of the professions. A 'model' represents a set of ideas derived from various fields of study which integrate elements of theory and practice. It influences the way people view their job and therefore how they work. This has implications for the consumer, namely the patient and his family. Their experiences of health care will depend upon the models (and hence practices) of the health workers they encounter.

This chapter summarizes some of the main approaches available in the care of the adult with acquired neurological brain damage. It concentrates on those which I have encountered when working with other professionals. There are also descriptions of some of the models based on these approaches. Later sections discuss several different professional practices and techniques. Similarities and differences are noted. The final part of the chapter looks at the implications for the patient and the professional both in hospital and in the community.

SOME APPROACHES TO HEALTH CARE

The Biomedical approach

This has traditionally been the basis for the practice of medicine in the Western world for the last few hundred years. It views human beings as biological entities comprised of cells, which make up tissues, which then make up organs, which in turn make up systems. All of these interact to create harmony or homeostasis. Biological homeostasis produces health but may be disrupted by trauma, malfunction or malformation. This leads to disease or medical conditions.

The biomedical model aims to cure or control disease by working on the physical symptoms. It evolved with the Renaissance when Descartes, a philosopher, proposed the concept of 'dualism'. Hitherto philosophical thinking had assumed that all actions were divinely controlled. With 'dualism', Descartes separated the mind from the body. He suggested that the mind could work on its own, free from external forces, whilst the body was like a machine made up of component parts.

These parts are the 'nuts and bolts' of the biomedical approach. The theory advocates studying the body by breaking it down into its component parts in order to identify and correct any malfunctioning of each one. Hence it is a 'reductionist' approach. It views reality as stable and measurable and favours objective, quantitative research under closely controlled experimental conditions. This allows results to be replicated and establishes scientific facts. Qualitative research using subjective data is considered unscientific and invalid.

The Neurodevelopmental Approach

The Neurodevelopmental Approach assumes that growth and change occur in recognized stages. Moreover they are caused by identifiable variables and move in a predictable direction. In the neurodevelopmental approach, the adult with acquired neurological impairment is thought to have regressed to a primitive neurodevelopmental level.

) Behaviourism

The Behaviourist Approach represents a theory of learning. It developed from research into stimulus response learning by Pavlov, Thorndike and Watson and, later, Skinner and others. The theory explains observable behaviour in terms of interaction with the environment. This provides stimuli to which the individual responds. Feedback allows him to appreciate the outcome of his response. Responses which are rewarded, or reinforced, become part of his behaviour. Those which are unsuccessful, or which produce unpleasant results, are discontinued.

Behaviour modification can be used both to teach a desirable behaviour or to remove an undesirable one. Fussey and Giles (1988) advocate the use of behavioural techniques for rehabilitation of the severely brain-injured adult. These, they say, allow therapists to manipulate the environment. This can be very helpful with an unmotivated patient or one who wants to achieve unrealistic goals.

The Humanist Approach

This is a strongly holistic approach which stresses the being as a whole and the way in which body and mind interact. It attaches great importance to the interaction of all the factors which make up an individual's experience – physical, social, psychological and so on. Personal experience and consciousness are crucial along with the right to choose. Factors which combine to create dysfunion in the individual include physical damage, lack of information preventing a correct choice, failure to achieve, lack of opportunity, poor self-esteem and so on.

Other approaches to health care

A variety of other approaches are available. They include the cognitive approach, the interactive approach and various problem-based models. They are not discussed in detail here but further information is available in Hagedorn (1992) and Pearson and Vaughan (1986). Atkinson *et al.* (1990) discuss some of these and other perspectives from a psychological point of view.

NURSING MODELS

Nursing theory today is governed by the concept of 'nursing models'. Developed to clarify the role of the nurse, a nursing model is a set of ideas about people and nursing. It can be used as a guide for the planning and delivery of nursing care (Aggleton and Chalmers, 1986). There are several different models available and also many different ways of classifying these. Riehl and Roy (1980) list a few under the headings of developmental models, system models and interaction models. Clarke (1991) adds some more but then gives a useful summary of the two most popular ones used in the UK in general adult nursing. These are Roper, Logan and Tierney's model of nursing and Orem's self-care model.

Roper, Logan and Tierney's model of nursing (1980)

This focuses on 12 activities of daily living (ADL), namely:

- maintaining a safe environment
- communicating
- breathing
- eating and drinking
- eliminating
- personal cleansing and cleaning
- controlling body temperature
- mobilizing
- working and playing
- expressing sexuality
- sleeping
- dying

Physical, psychological, sociocultural, environmental and politico-economic factors affect these ADL along with the individual's age. The nurse assesses each one on a dependence-independence continuum. She then sets goals and plans and evaluates care by focussing on those ADL for which the individual needs help.

Clarke (1991) maintains that the Roper, Logan and Tierney model is the most popular one in the UK at present. There are several reasons for this. It does not use jargon and is easy to apply. It is appropriate for a wide variety of people with physical health problems. More over it ensures reasonably comprehensive nursing care and is simple.

Orem's self-care model (1980)

This model revolves around the concept of self-care. There are six universal self-care demands, namely:

- adequate intake of air, water and food;
- adequate excretion of waste products;
- balance between rest and activity;
- optimizing social interaction and solitude;
- avoiding and preventing hazards to life and well-being;
- avoiding stress by feeling and being normal.

Illness involves additional factors which are called health deviation self-care needs. These relate to changes in body structure, physical function and behaviour. Using Orem's model, the nurse identifies health deviation self-care needs and universal self-care deficits. She then assesses why the patient cannot meet self-care demands. Goals of care are prioritized, but formulated and shared with the patient and his family. Their role is considered vital in achieving a return to self-care. Thus the model contrasts with Roper *et al.*'s model because it focuses on the patient's own role. Clarke (1991) says that it is a particularly good model for rehabilitation. It concentrates on identifying outcomes of care rather than on nursing interventions.

Models are used along with the nursing process (see Chapter 4). By following the four steps of the nursing process, namely assessment, planning, implementation and evaluation, the models guide the way nursing is delivered.

Organization of nursing care on the ward

Although nursing models affect the delivery of nursing care another factor is also relevant. This is the organization of nursing care on the ward. Nursing in hospital can be organized in different ways. Task assignment, team nursing, patient assignment and primary nursing are the main methods which have been used. The first is now thought to be more-or-less outdated. However the second approach, **team nursing**, is used in many hospitals today. In this, groups of patients in the ward, whose beds are near to one another, are cared for by a team of nurses who are a subgroup of the total ward staff.

In the third method, **patient assignment**, each nurse is allocated a group of patients and is responsible for their nursing care. This method is used in the community by district nurses. The last method, **primary nursing**, is now the method chosen

by many units in the UK. Each nurse has a number of patients
for whom she is responsible. The primary nurse interviews the
patient to obtain the history, records the nursing assessment
and writes the care plan. When she is away from the ward, she
hands over to another nurse who gives nursing care according
to the care plan until the primary nurse returns. The primary
nurse is responsible and accountable for the patient throughout
the stay in hospital even when she is not on duty. This ensures
continuity of care. Other nurses who help in the patient's care
are called 'associates'. The ward sister acts as a coordinator
designating who is the primary nurse and who are the associate
nurses for each individual patient.

PHYSIOTHERAPY TECHNIQUES

In physiotherapy the principles behind rehabilitation and treatment techniques have changed considerably over the last 30
years or so. Some of these are complementary whilst others
conflict directly with each other. Lynch and Grisogono (1991)
explain the concepts of each method. The following sections
summarize their remarks.

The compensatory method

This was the traditional method of treatment for the hemiplegic
patient. Aiming to restore independence as soon as possible, it
involved strengthening and stretching exercises for the affected
arm and leg. It also allowed the patient to use his unaffected
side to walk and move about. Lynch and Grisogono (1991) paint
a desperate picture of this now outdated type of treatment.
Over-compensation by the normal side left the patient with no
real control of his movements. Sticks, tripods and quadropods
allowed him to walk slowly by dragging his affected leg along.
However he had no balance and was therefore unable to carry
out simple activities without falling.

   Lynch and Grisogono (1991) point out that it is spasticity and
not muscle weakness which is the biggest problem in hemiplegia. Strengthening exercises are inappropriate because they
inevitably make the spasticity worse.

Conductive education

This is a treatment pioneered by Professor Andreas Peto in Hungary. It is a highly structured and formal system, originally used with cerebral palsied children. Now it is also applied to adult neurological impairment. It involves analysing functional tasks, for example the series of movements needed to walk. The patient is then taught how to perform these movements. Consistent practice involves the use of 'rhythmic intention'. This encourages the patient to say out loud what movement he is about to do and then count aloud as he performs it. Thus each action is given its own rhythm. Treatment programmes are intensive, tailored to suit each individual and involve reasonable goals.

Motor learning programme

This developed in Australia in the late 1970s. It involves teaching the patient specific functional tasks by breaking these down in to their constituent parts. The patient then masters the different movements involved bit by bit. Lynch and Grisogono (1991) point out that this approach requires good balance and awareness. It is inappropriate for those with severe neurological damage.

The Bobath concept

Berta Bobath, a physiotherapist, developed the Bobath Method in the late 1940s when she worked with cerebral palsied children. Later she extended her work to adult hemiplegic patients. Her techniques continue to evolve but her basic principles remain the same. Hence the treatment is called the Bobath concept, modifying itself over time, rather than the Bobath method, which implies a fixed programme.

The Bobath concept is a bilateral approach to the treatment of hemiplegia or spasticity. The two main principles of treatment are:

1. inhibition of unwanted muscle patterns, namely flexion in the upper limb and extension in the lower limb;
2. facilitation of the automatic reactions of righting, equilibrium and protective extension.

The patient is positioned in a way that inhibits the development of abnormal reflexes and the unwanted muscle patterns described above. This reduces abnormal muscle tone and allows him to re-learn normal movement patterns. In addition, correct handling, use of sensory stimulation and use of key control points on the body facilitate correct movement. The concepts of righting and equilibrium reactions are considered vital. Treatment aims to re-establish these. Both sides of the body are used as patient and therapist work through a developmental sequence (lying, 'all-fours', trunk control, sitting, standing, weight transfer, stepping and walking).

Thus, with guidance, the patient learns how to use his affected arm and leg confidently for normal activities such as balancing, walking, dressing and eating. Abnormal spastic reactions which would interfere with these are reduced.

The Johnstone concept of rehabilitation

This is a method for the treatment of stroke developed in the 1970s by the British physiotherapist Margaret Johnstone. Like Bobath, she advocates inhibiting the abnormal patterns of movement associated with spasticity to allow postural control to be re-established. Correct positioning is combined with exercise routines performed by the patient. Inflatable pressure splints are used to help hold the patient's leg and arm against spastic forces.

OCCUPATIONAL THERAPY TECHNIQUES

Occupational therapists use a variety of techniques based on one or many of the approaches outlined at the beginning of this chapter. The Bobath concept and conductive education have already been discussed. Others include the following:

Proprioceptive neuromuscular facilitation

This technique was initially developed by Herman Kabat and expanded by Margaret Knott and Dorothy Voss throughout the 1950s, 1960s and 1970s. It emphasizes the use of resisted movement, manual contacts and voice tones during treatment. These combine to reinforce desired movement patterns.

The Rood approach

This is named after an American, Margaret Rood, who was both a physical therapist and an occupational therapist. She used sensory stimulation to modify motor patterns in stroke patients. She maintained that if correct sensory stimulation is applied to sensory receptors, then a motor response could be elicited as a reflex. This could then be re-established as a normal movement pattern. Many kinds of different tactile stimulation are used – brushing, icing, tapping, pressure and stretch reflexes.

Other techniques

Other techniques used in occupational therapy include behaviour modification, perceptual training, memory training, work retraining and resettlement, reality orientation, problem solving, providing aids and home adaptations, prescribing and providing orthoses, adapting activities and apparatuses, counselling and many more, Further information is available in Hagedorn (1992) and in the well-known occupational therapy textbooks such as *Willard and Spackman's Occupational Therapy* (Hopkins and Smith, 1988).

Occupational therapy models

Like nursing, occupational therapy also uses different models, Hagedorn (1992) maintains that the use of models in the profession is more fashionable in the US than in the UK. She describes three, namely Gary Kielhofner's model of human occupation, Kathleen Reed's adaptation through occupations model and Anne Cronin Mosey's adaptive skills model. All these stress the importance of occupations in the life of the individual and their consequent value as therapy.

TECHNIQUES USED IN CLINICAL PSYCHOLOGY

The clinical psychologist working with the neurologically damaged adult may used a number of techniques depending upon the patient and his difficulties. Fussey and Giles (1988) advocate use of behaviour modification. This involves setting a precise behavioural objective for the patient to achieve. Firstly a positive reinforcer or reward is established often as part of a contract with the patient. It may be food, drink, a privilege, an enjoyable activity and so on. The reward is given following successful performance. Some behaviour modification programmes operate by providing opportunities for the behaviour to occur. They may also prompt, shape or cue the response. Once the behaviour, after consistent reinforcement, becomes established, the reward may be gradually withdrawn.

Other techniques used by the clinical psychologist include counselling, relaxation techniques, problem solving training, memory and perceptual training and many more.

SPEECH AND LANGUAGE THERAPY TECHNIQUES

For the adult with acquired neurological damage, speech and language therapists concentrate on the areas of communication and swallowing. They use a variety of techniques to treat dysphasia, dysphagia, and dysarthria. Those used in **dysphasia** are based on seven different approaches (Howard and Hatfield, 1987) summarized as follows:

The didactic approach. This involves re-teaching language using a number of practical methods. It descends from the language therapy of the nineteenth and early twentieth century – using clinical intuition, common sense and the traditional methods of teaching reading, writing and grammar to children and non-brain-damaged foreigners.

Behaviour modification. This, too, involves re-teaching language using the principles drawn from behaviourist psychology described above.

The stimulation approach. This was developed by Joseph Wepman and Hildred Schuell, American therapists of the 1940s and 1950s. It provides appropriate stimulation to enable the aphasic to regain access to language abilities that remain largely intact but unusable.

The reorganization of function approach. This derives from work during and after the Second World War by Alexander Luria, a Soviet neurologist. It views language as a number of quasi-independent physiological subsystems. Therapy involves learning to use intact subsystems in different ways to bypass those that are impaired.

The pragmatic approach. This stresses communication as a whole rather than language. Therapy concentrates on developing good use of unimpaired abilities (for example non-verbal skills) to compensate for the language problem.

The neo-classical approach. This developed in the 1960s along with neuropsychology. It uses relatively intact abilities of the aphasic to support the uncovering of inaccessible language abilities.

The neurolinguistic school. This incorporates sophisticated linguistic theories into therapy.

The cognitive neuropsychology approach. This uses theories of modern cognitive neuropsychology and involves complex models of language processing.

In the field of **dysphagia**, treatment techniques follow a biomedical approach. The component parts of the swallowing system are assessed (see Chapter 4). Treatment then works on those parts that are impaired, for example tongue action, the triggering of the swallowing reflex and so on. Some methods aim to help the patient compensate for impaired ability – for example posture may be modified to reduce the risk of aspiration.

Similar strategies are used in the treatment of **dysarthria**. The component parts of the vocal tract are assessed (see Chapter 4). Treatment then involves working on these to improve their function. There are also ways of getting the patient to compensate for his impaired abilities. Specific techniques such as proprioceptive neuromuscular facilitation can also be incorporated into the treatment of dysarthria.

Speech and language therapists are also involved in providing appropriate communication aids. In addition they may use more holistic approaches in techniques such as counselling and relaxation.

TECHNIQUES USED IN DIETETICS

There are many reasons why a patient cannot maintain an adequate nutritional intake. A poor or absent swallowing reflex, mental illness, lack of strength and control in chewing and drinking, malabsorption, poor dentures, physical disability and pain, and increased loss from diarrhoea are just a few. The dietician gives concrete, physical support by adding nutritional density to normal meals, especially where patients need a puréed diet. She may also provide supplementary food and drinks which contain the complete range of vitamins and minerals. Nasogastric and gastrostomy feeds may be prescribed as the only source of nutrition or as supplements to an inadequate intake by mouth. Where the gut is inaccessible or malfunctioning, intravenous nutrition may be used as a permanent or temporary measure. A combination of feeding routes may be used to maintain adequate nutrition.

Another type of intervention from the dietician includes informal discussion, for example when liaising with other staff and when talking to patients and carers themselves.

AREAS OF OVERLAP

The above sections illustrate that the practices of the different professions overlap in several ways. Many use techniques which originate from behaviourism. Other strategies are more holistic whilst yet others have their origins in a biomedical approach to health care. Certain practices are common to some professions. The Bobath concept is an example of this as it may be used by both physiotherapists and occupational therapists. Similarly, proprioceptive neuromuscular facilitation may be used by both these groups and by speech and language therapists.

Another example of an activity common to most professional groups is counselling. Counselling is 'the means by which one person helps another to clarify their life situation and to decide upon further lines of action' (Burnard, 1989; p. 2). Smyth (1990) observes that this is one of the many common areas in which different professions have developed separate expertise. Those with the most expertise in this area are probably the clinical psychologist and the social worker, although others also have a basic knowledge of what it involves and how to do it.

Whatever the level of expertise, each profession uses their counselling skills in a way that relates to their own profession. The nurse, for example, may use it when coping with dying or bereaved people whilst the physiotherapist may use it to help patients regain their motivation for rehabilitation. These are simply two examples. Numerous others from all the professions could be listed. The crucial point for all non-specialist counsellors is to know when the patient and his family need access to higher levels of expertise. Appropriate referral to the clinical psychologist, for example, may be required.

Counselling forms part of the skills which are shared between professional groups. Core skills, on the other hand, are the basic components of practice by which they differ. Analysis of the textbooks of individual professions reveals a strong emphasis on developing specialist core skills. Indeed it is these which set the professions apart from one another. Core skills are therefore considered important because they strengthen the importance of the individual profession. They are the emblems by which it is recognized and which give it status.

In the context of teamwork, however, shared skills, can be equally important. They, too, should receive high prominence and status because they provide a common foundation on which individuals can begin to work with each other. Recognizing and sharing common knowledge like this can result in establishing trust and good working relations. This can lead the way to sharing specialist knowledge in a friendly, non-threatening manner. Professional jealousies, which merely limit team work and efficient patient care, are reduced.

IMPLICATIONS FOR THE PATIENT

The above sections show that in each profession, a wide variety of treatment techniques are available. These are based upon different approaches which have developed as individual professions have evolved. Such variety carries potential disadvantages. In hospital, for example, one professional may follow one type of model whilst another may favour a different one. This may produce conflict in the rationale behind treatment, creating different goals. The end result is a disjointed programme causing confusion for the patient and his family.

The plethora of approaches has further implications for the patient. Without being a specialist in each profession, he cannot possible be aware of all the techniques available. Hence he may expect one sort of treatment because that is the only one he knows. This is usually the old, biomedically-based, traditional method which has passed out of fashion. It is also the one by which the professional is recognized in the community at large. The use of a 'ball for squeezing' as part of physiotherapy treatment is a frequent example. Relatives often give patients items to hold with their affected hand and tell them to squeeze it. They interpret a tightening of hand grip as increased and therefore improved muscle power. In reality this behaviour on the part of the patient can merely be a sign of increased spasticity. Hence requests by relatives and by doctors telling the patient to 'squeeze my hand' may be inappropriate. They may simply produce tightening of the finger flexors and an inability to release an object when it is grasped (Bukowski *et al.*, 1986). This response hampers the return of normal muscle tone which is necessary for starting to re-learn normal movement.

Without up-to-date theoretical knowledge, both patient and family may think that the professional is not doing her job properly. They may assume, without even knowing it, that a biomedical approach, the basis of medicine for many years, governs all therapy as well. If this fails to materialize, complaints to other staff, ill-feeling, and lack of cooperation and motivation for treatment may ensure. One way of circumventing the problem is for the professional to realize why relatives expect a certain form of treatment. She can then begin to explain, sensitively and diplomatically why a different approach is needed and what this is.

Examples like this illustrate how the prominence of the biomedical model can colour the attitudes and the perceptions of the public. The model has traditionally governed health care and is the one which receives the most publicity. Both the British government, and the media, continue to advertise a 'cure rather than care' approach. They pay attention to recovery from definable diseases by the treatment of physical deficits.

This may be for historical reasons, other more holistic approaches being less fashionable. Hence the media give time and space to reports of high-tech surgery such as heart transplants and kidney transplants. Recovery in these areas is measured in compartmentalized understandable physical terms. The staff who work in the specialized units enjoy high status. Moreover government finance for these specialities is more forthcoming than it is for those fields where recovery is impossible – for example for the adult with Alzheimer's disease or motor neurone disease. The perceived status of those who work with the demented or with the elderly multiply neurologically impaired may be lower than the status of specialists whose goal is to cure.

IMPLICATIONS FOR THE PROFESSIONAL

The existence and use of different approaches has various implications for the professional working in a team. Firstly she needs to be aware of the rationale behind the treatment techniques of her colleagues. Without this she will not have a full grasp of *why* certain practices are followed. This lack of understanding will have a negative effect on overall patient care because it leaves people working in isolation from each other. The therapist therefore needs to seek out her colleagues and *ask* for information as well as providing it.

In hospital, this can be done informally, during daily working contact. In the community, it can be more difficult because meetings between team members may be infrequent. Here, persistence is the key, by phone if necessary, despite the initial difficulties in tracking someone down at a convenient time. In the ideal world, specific multidisciplinary in-service training offers invaluable benefits and this will be discussed further in Chapter 6.

There are other implications for the professional. If at all possible, all those who are working with the patient should try to agree on the model they wish to follow. In the words of one nursing textbook 'the whole basis of multidisciplinary team work is the bringing together of people who are able to practise from different model bases acquired through professional training' (Pearson and Vaughan, 1986, p. 46).

Agreeing on a model may be difficult for the newly-qualified fledgling therapist whose status amongst the other workers is low. She may be struggling to develop her own core skills and have little time or energy to think about the practices of those about her. Liaison like this may be just as difficult for the junior hospital nurse who has no influence and simply uses the model currently in vogue on her ward. However 5 or 10 minutes spent on discovering aspects of the treatment of the other professions, the ward organization (do they follow a team nursing or a primary nursing approach?) and so on, may pay dividends in the long run.

The information gained may enable the therapist to establish who to report to on the ward, and the best way of doing this. Such efforts also increase contact with other staff and help to build up relations on a friendly, informal basis. Consider the possible reaction of the person who is asked by someone else a little bit about their job. It is surprisingly easy to assume that everyone knows what you are trying to achieve. It may come as a pleasant surprise to discover that others do not know as much as you do and that they are genuinely interested in hearing about your expertise.

A further implication for the professional involves the treatment she decides to initiate. Some techniques despite their acclaimed advantages, may be totally useless because of the environment in which they are applied. Hagedorn (1992) points out that neurodevelopmental techniques such as the Bobath method, Rood technique or proprioceptive neuromusucalr facilitation have disappointing results unless used intensively, skilfully and correctly by all members of the treatment team. She adds that most neurodevelopmental techniques require special training for effective use.

There is, in addition, the thorny question of the efficacy of treatment. The paramedical professions are still struggling to prove to others, especially doctors, that they are doing some good. Evidence is hardly encouraging. Fussey and Giles (1988) report studies comparing the effectiveness of neurodevelopmental approaches such as the Bobath concept with the training of functional skills. No significant difference was found between the two, even when the neurodevelopmental treatment involved many more therapy hours (Stern *et al.*, 1970; Logigan *et al.*, 1983; Lord and Hall, 1986).

Allen *et al.* (1988) also question the effectiveness of therapy. After summarizing the main points drawn from reviews of the effectiveness of therapy for stroke, they conclude that intensity of therapy makes no difference. They say a therapist can see a patient for only 3–5% of her waking time each week (Wade *et al.*, 1984). Family and nurse are the vital helpers. For speech and language therapy they maintain that the optimal type and amount of therapy, the criteria for selecting patients, and the extent of any benefits are unknown. They do admit, however, that some patients given large amounts of therapy tailored to their problem probably do benefit (Howard *et al.*, 1985).

My own clinical impression is that professionals unfamiliar with the theory and rationale behind any technique, proven or otherwise, are reluctant to practise it because they do not see the results. They do not know the long-term advantages and disadvantages of pursuing a specific approach because they do not have the detailed theoretical knowledge necessary to understand why something is done. Therefore their motivation to provide continuity of treatment is low. They need to see the immediate benefits if they are to carry out advice rigorously.

If this is the case, then perhaps the Bobath concept, or proprioceptive neuromuscular facilitation, used in isolation only when the therapist is on duty is a waste of time. Such methods may be better suited to a unified setting, such as a head injury unit. Here staff have to care for the same type of client group and in-service training may be easier (see Chapter 6). Similarly the Bobath concept and, for example, cognitive neuropsychology in speech and language therapy may be inappropriate in the patient's home – *unless* the patient and family are able to carry out the techniques effectively. No doubt these are controversial remarks with which many will disagree. The overall conclusion, however, is that staff in-service training is of crucial importance (see Chapter 6).

A frequent complaint from people working in health care is that members of other professions fail to carry out their advice and recommendations. This happens even in those units which profess to follow a team approach. The complainant is often exasperated because she knows that her treatment would work if only the others would back it up. Examples of this are the use of the Bobath concept by physiotherapists, advice on safe swallowing procedures from the speech and language therapist, dressing practice by the occupational therapist and so on. The problem seems to be a mismatch in the perceptions of different professions about the importance of each other's work. This may arise because each operates different principles and conflicting models.

Hence agreeing on a model has a further benefit. It ensures the best chance of continuity of treatment. Indeed staff who do adopt a similar approach tend to understand each other better. For example the social worker and the clinical psychologist may work well together because they follow a humanistic approach without realizing it.

Agreeing on a model, however, relies upon other people knowing what approach they are already following. My clinical experience suggests that many professionals follow an eclectic approach without realizing it. They use bits and pieces from various models depending upon the needs of the patient. This is particularly true for those who undertook training some years ago. Often they just 'do the job' (and do it well) without thinking about the theory behind it. When asked about the model or models they use they are unable to say.

Contemporary students voice the reason for this when they say that theory at college bears little relation to what they experience in practice. This observation is not confined to one profession. It has been mentioned by nursing students on the ward, and by paramedical students both in hospital or in the community as part of their clinical placement.

There is nothing wrong with an eclectic approach like this. Indeed there is no right answer to the treatment of patients' problems (Hagedorn, 1992). The important thing is for individuals to know why they choose to work in a particular way and to discover what makes the other professions tick as well. This sharing of knowledge will improve communication and therefore enhance patient care. New therapists are particularly vulnerable because they may enthusiastically adopt one approach at the expense of all others. Coming straight from college, they may favour the most recent model which is the flavour of the month there and promoted exclusively. Old hands in the job, on the other hand, may adopt the attitude 'we've seen it all before'. In other words, theories have come and gone and their basic practices have not changed. Nevertheless it is still beneficial to know why one works in a particular way.

An example of this is in the field of speech and language therapy. Here the cognitive neuropsychological approach to aphasia therapy is sacrosanct. It is also the most recent. It requires 'general linguistics' expertise to operate, forming part of the aphasia therapist's core skills. However it is not appropriate for all dysphasic patients. Furthermore it is highly complex, treats a very narrow area of communication and probably offers little to the nurse who has to communicate with the patient on the ward. Thus the speech and language therapist may need to adopt a more eclectic approach – especially if she wants other staff to understand what she is trying to do.

There is a final important point to end this chapter on approaches and models. The traditional biomedical model is not always appropriate in the care of the neurologically damaged adult (see Chapter 2). A holistic approach, for example, is crucial in the care of the dying patient. Unfortunately this is rarely taught at medical school (Baldwin and Hopcroft, 1987), although some doctors have at least identified this as a problem.

The Independent newspaper (14 April 1992) reported the feelings of Dr Nicki Henderson who developed ovarian cancer. Her personal experience of treatment left a strong impression. Doctors, she maintains, are just not equipped to deal with the patient's psychological and emotional stress – 'doctors just don't have the right training'. In such cases, the traditional biomedical model, with its objective, scientific, quantitative methods may have little to offer.

There are implications for the rest of the team working with the adult with acquired neurological brain damage. Therapists and nurses who follow a holistic approach should not be put off by medical dogma and its pursuit for objectivity. Their own holistic methods are equally valid and can be used as the basis for research. This is particularly true where the aim is, for example, improvement in the patient's quality of remaining life rather than cure of a terminal illness.

6

Training and education for teamwork

This chapter investigates various aspects of training and education in medicine, nursing, physiotherapy, occupational therapy, speech and language therapy, clinical psychology, dietetics, and social work. Features common to the professions and those which set them apart are discussed. After this, there are suggestions about how training could be modified to encourage greater teamwork. This includes both student training and in-service training on the job. Further discussion of running workshops in a hospital highlight features based on clinical experience. Following this there is an outline of certain nursing procedures which are important for any therapist working with the adult with acquired neurological brain damage. Legal and financial implications are discussed.

FEATURES COMMON TO THE PROFESSIONS

The professions discussed in this book all have certain characteristics in common with regard to education and career development. Firstly, much of the student's work involves practical 'hands on' training. This usually takes place under the guidance and supervision of a fully-qualified, senior individual working in the field. Furthermore all the professions have their own characteristic career structures. These have developed over time as each one has evolved.

On the whole the newly qualified nurse, paramedic, social worker and clinical psychologist spend about 2–3 years in their first post, gaining general experience. This forms the basis on which they can begin to specialize in a chosen area. After specialization over a number of years, some turn to teaching posts, others to managerial positions. The number of years this takes usually depends upon the profession involved and the individual's experience and circumstances.

Training for a specialization in hospital medicine, can take up to about 10 years (or more, depending upon the availability of posts). Specialization in other careers tends to take less time. Furthermore a variety of ranks exist throughout the professions. Nurses and speech and language therapists, for example, achieve certain grades as they progress up the ladder. Physiotherapists, occupational therapists and dieticians, on the other hand, have different titles (Basic Grade, Senior I, Senior II and so on).

These similarities and differences in training and education have implications for the patient. Firstly, he is likely to encounter a fair number of students during his care, both in hospital and in the community. In my experience, professionals, particularly doctors, fail to address the use of student assistance in clinical work. They neither introduce the student to the patient nor, in some cases, obtain his consent to student examination and treatment. Nevertheless these are basic requirements contributing to quality of care.

The widely different career structures have further implications for the patient. He is confronted with a vast array of people of various ranks, doing different jobs, each progressing up their separate career ladder. Confusion reigns about their titles, ranks, and statuses. Uniforms, or lack of them, create further uncertainty (see Chapter 2). For this reason it is useful for all staff to have a basic knowledge of other people's career structures and ranks. Taking the time to explain these can be a great help to the bewildered patient and his relatives. It also has further advantages. It allows individuals to appreciate the slot their colleagues occupy in their own profession. Such understanding may allow them to recognize more easily the pressures their colleagues are under – and perhaps empathize with them.

PROMOTING TEAMWORK WITHIN EDUCATION
AND TRAINING

Student training

The basic core skills of a profession are learnt during the student years. These are the primary components of professional practice. The nurse, for example, learns how to perform a nursing assessment, record temperature, pulse and heart rate, perform a drug round and so on. The occupational therapist, on the other hand, learns how to do a standardized test of perception and to conduct a home visit. These are only two examples. There are numerous others which differentiate the professions from one another.

However there is little emphasis, during training, on learning how to blend skills and work as a member of a team. The problem is one of sharing knowledge. This is particularly difficult when each profession has its own separate training system (Smyth, 1990). At present, what tends to happen is the occasional 'guest speaker' appearance during a lecture course. A member of a different profession may be invited to give a talk on a particular topic or provide one or two lectures. Thus, for example, a physiotherapist might be asked to talk to speech and language therapists about cerebral palsy.

However the 'guest speaker' arrangement, however informal or *ad hoc*, is important in learning about each others' roles. Indeed for students, meeting a member of a different profession may benefit teamwork. Lorenz and Pichert (1986) found this when they investigated the training of medical students. They looked at the multidisciplinary training of students in diabetes care. They found that the students were more willing to share responsibility with a nurse when they thought they had learned that topic, during a seminar, from a nurse. The authors suggest that the medical students' experience in observing nurses at work may have been important in influencing attitudes towards team care.

Mody and Nagai (1990) also highlight the benefits of joint training and education between professions. They describe greater levels of trust between occupational therapists and speech and language therapists in the area of dysphagia. This occurred when the two professions developed competency standards together and jointly allocated who should see a patient with dysphagia and when. The net result was that the two professions became less territorial.

Other authors have considered the topic of joint training in the care of the neurologically disabled. Madsen *et al.* (1988) discuss a pilot project for educating students. Their work took place at an interdisciplinary clinic for adults with neurological impairment. They suggest that before clinical services can operate together successfully, there needs to be an integrated academic curriculum for training. Henderson *et al.* (1990) also have something to say about training. They discuss the possibility of the nurse learning the skills of other professionals. They suggest, for this, a national postbasic course in rehabilitation. The nurse would neither usurp the role of the other professions nor take on their unwanted tasks. Henderson *et al.* argue instead that this extra specialist expertise would enable the nurse to become a more effective member of the team.

The literature summarized above has implications for the training of paramedical and nursing students. Perhaps teamwork between these professions would improve if they underwent some of their basic education together. This novel approach is used already in training occupational therapists and physiotherapists at the University of East Anglia in the UK (Routledge and Willson, 1992). Further ideas on joint education and training are discussed below.

(a) Joint lectures

Joint lectures for students of different professions already occur in some training schools. The teaching of basic medical topics such as anatomy, neurology, and psychology may be delivered to more than one profession at the same time. Other more specific subjects could be added – in particular counselling, an important part of nursing, physiotherapy, occupational therapy and speech and language therapy (cf. Thurgood, 1992). All these professions have developed their expertise in this area separately (Burnard, 1989). Similarly team-building exercises offer further opportunities for sharing and supporting one another, removing defensive barriers and establishing closer working relationships.

Another important topic could be shared by students of different disciplines. This concerns 'models of practice'. These act as a framework guiding different professional practices (see Chapter 5). Lecturers and tutors from the different disciplines could combine to offer a cohesive package on the subject. Several benefits might accrue from this policy. Firstly, students might gain a greater understanding of why some professions work in a particular way. Furthermore being taught by someone who does a different, but related job might enhance working relations and teamwork after qualification. Indeed the chances of this might increase if the students actually saw how their own tutors had managed to combine their expertise – even though they belonged to different professions.

(b) Joint practical work

Joint education could be extended to include practical issues as well. Students of different professions could be asked to complete a short, joint project as part of their clinical placement. This need be neither detailed nor time-consuming. It could simply be something which aims to get the students talking and working together. Topics of joint interest, for example, could be given to a pair of students who attended the same location as part of their practical training. After their joint investigation, they could then offer a short presentation to their peers on the subject.

An example of such a project might be joint assessment by a physiotherapist and a speech and language therapist of a patient with a poor chest condition and swallowing problems. Both professions are concerned with topics such as the anatomy and physiology of respiration, posture, sitting balance and so on. Yet they approach these from different viewpoints. A joint project on a real case like this might enable students to understand more easily the role and contribution of the other profession. Another example of joint projects like this is home visits between social work students and occupational therapy students. A simple form of joint record keeping (see Chapter 4) could be included. This would encourage teamwork even further, concentrating upon the patient's needs rather than on what individuals do separately to help a patient.

Dittmar (1989) points out that such collaboration rarely occurs. Therefore students of different professions have little chance to appreciate the viewpoints of others. This is essential

if they are to work successfully in a team after they have qualified. Thus today's insular training contributes to defensive barriers which prevent people from working together.

The suggestions above, of course, require a great deal of
practical organization. Student's clinical placements would need
to overlap at least a little (this does actually happen in some
hospitals). Their tutors and clinical supervisors would need to
guide their projects and provide support. This presupposes
that these same tutors are willing to work together themselves,
coordinating their courses and student training schedules. Such
a mammoth task could not be achieved easily. It might require
a joint introductory seminar from the two tutors themselves as
well as good working relations between the clinical supervisors
already working in the two disciplines (further evidence of the
need to work together).

Perhaps, however, it could be done on a pilot basis with two
tutors coordinating student contract and work in one location.
Benefits and problems could then be discussed and attempts
made to circumvent these on subsequent occasions. This kind
of joint contact and training will obviously work more easily at
those schools, colleges and universities where the two professions already exist side by side.

Joint projects, such as those suggested above, might have a
further benficial spin-off. Frequently students in all the professions encounter tutors and lecturers with, what they perceive
as, little relevant recent clinical experience. Hence they complain that what they are being taught in college has little relevance to what they experience out in the field during their
placements. The ongoing dispute over the status of the National
Health Service is an example of this in the UK. At work, departments are fighting to keep staff, maintain their autonomy as
hospitals become independent 'trusts' and survive within an
increasingly competitive market. The student, on the other
hand, learns about assessment, treatment, management and
evaluation of specific patients. She receives little information
on management and policies. Nevertheless these matters will
largely dictate whether she can carry out her job when she
qualifies and starts work.

If tutors from different professions combine to organize training together, they may be forced to face the problems encountered by those working in the field. They can learn from this

and appreciate what it is like outside the protective confines of college. They may then be able to adopt a more sympathetic attitude to their students.

IN-SERVICE TRAINING

Training and education should not be confined to the student during her pre-qualification years. It can and does take place for those already working. There are study days and courses for all types of staff both in hospital and in the community. Nurses may attend, for example, courses on primary nursing, the treatment of pressure sores and so on. Physiotherapists may have training about developments in chest care and clinical psychologists may attend study days devoted to advances in cognitive neuropsychology. These are only a few examples and there are numerous others. They tend to be organized by a particular profession for its own members. Staff from other disciplines do not usually attend because they do not have the specialist interest in the topic to be discussed.

Other courses which are offered are multidisciplinary. Sometimes they revolve around the management of a particular disorder. During a study day on motor neurone disease, for example, there may be contributions on various aspects of the disease from a representative of the Motor Neurone Disease Association, the district nurse, the social worker, the neurologist, the physiotherapist and the speech and language therapist, to name just a few. This type of in-service training offers a valuable insight into the multiplicity of problems of the disease and the ways in which they can be handled effectively.

There should be more opportunity and encouragement to attend and contribute to joint workshops like these. Smyth (1990) observes that professions can often combine in their training needs. Nurses and physiotherapists, for example, may learn a lot from each other in attending a joint course on the fractured neck of femur. Similarly physiotherapists, nurses and speech and language therapists can learn about each others' roles in courses on swallowing problems in the neurologically impaired. Finally, multidisciplinary research, such as that established in Aberdeen in the UK (Chesson, 1992), is a further way of promoting teamwork.

Running joint multidisciplinary workshops in a hospital

Several points have come to light during my experience of running joint multidisciplinary courses, study days or workshops. These can be discussed under the headings of, content, manner of presentation, and participants.

Content

Staff of one profession do not respond favourably to dry theoretical facts delivered by a member of another profession. For one thing they tend to forget them. Such 'dead knowledge' keeps no better than fish (Whitehead, 1922). For another they often seem to infer that the information is not directly relevant because it was not part of their own core education. There are other matters related to content. Participants do not want any workshop to intrude too much into their working routine. If the course is an hour or so, or even a half day, they already have enough to do and think about at work. They do not welcome an extra burden placed on their remaining mental energy. This simply causes extra stress. Hence the content of in-service training workshops needs to be practical rather than theoretical. Furthermore it needs to be directly relevant to the needs of the people who attend. This emphasis ensures that the participants do not fall asleep. It also encourages motivation and participation. Finally it gives them the best chance of remembering something which has been said.

Manner of presentation

The way information is given affects the success of the workshop and whether advice is remembered afterwards. Colleagues from other professions and myself have agreed that 'simulation' has been our most successful technique so far. This involves the use of props to help participants experience sensory or motor deprivation. We have also used role play. One of several methods of experiential learning listed by Burnard (1990), this involves setting up an imagined and possible situation, and acting out that situation. It also involves reflection and feedback to allow learning. Examples of simulation and role play appear in the literature. Bishop *et al.* (1990) describe a student group of Registered Nurses for the Mentally Handicapped who spent 24 hours living like their mentally handicapped clients in wheelchairs. They recount their experiences and feel the exercise heightened their awareness of what it feels like to be disabled.

We have used techniques like these to give informal workshops on the management of swallowing difficulties in patients with a stroke. This enabled the participants to experience what it felt like not to be able to eat and swallow normally. However, over time, we realized that simulation and role play have to be introduced and managed with care. This is because those who come to a workshop do so to learn and not to receive therapy (Burnard, 1990). Therefore they are reluctant to adopt the role of the patient. This reluctance is quite understandable and, if ignored, may breed resentment, hostility and non-cooperation.

To reduce the feeling of threat, my colleagues and I elected first to model some of the activities we wanted the others to do. This involved one of us acting as a patient. The physiotherapist positioned this person in a chair in a way that would cause maximum discomfort and postural problems if it were allowed to continue for any length of time. 'Favourite' postures included sitting slumped to one side, with a spastic right hemiplegia, the right arm extended and hanging over the side of the chair, the right leg extended outwards, the hips near the front edge of the chair, and the head tilted to the right. Although this was artificial, it did reflect the positions in which many patients end up whilst sitting.

In addition, the 'patient' did not talk throughout the interaction. This also often happens in real life. This person, the 'patient', was then fed by another of us, using all the wrong techniques (too fast, large unwieldy cutlery, too much at once, talking at the same time, and so on). The food included hospital mousse and, later, cake. Drinks from a beaker with a spout and/or a tumbler were also given. The effects on the participants were dramatic. They readily identified negative factors which they had noticed. They also offered ways of altering these.

Modelling proved a useful way of breaking the ice. After witnessing a scene such as that above and discussing it, participants are quite prepared to have a go at other sorts of simulation and role play themselves. Sessions have been fun. We have also linked the topics covered in the workshop to current patients on the ward. This has made the training directly relevant to the experience of the participants. They have found this particularly useful. Furthermore we, too, have learnt from their comments and ideas. This two-way transfer of information in a non-threatening environment has been vital in maintaining people's interest, motivation and cooperation.

The participants

Another important aspect for in-service training concerns the participants themselves. Therapists often try to organize informal training for nursing staff on a hospital ward. This may relate to a variety of topics – the Bobath concept, dressing techniques, and speech and language disorders to name just a few. Often, painstaking preparation meets with failure simply because staff fail to attend. This may happen for a variety of reasons. Shortage of staff to cover for the ward during the workshop, indifference, and reluctance to accept 'non-nursing' information are just some of these. This can be particularly frustrating for the therapist. She may feel disillusioned and disheartened because her honest attempts to share her expertise and thereby improve patient care are ignored.

A further problem is the rank of the staff who attend. The following points are based on my own clinical experience. Ideally, therapists would like all the regular ward staff to come, particularly the senior staff. It is they who guide ward policy. Therefore they are the people to target if there is to be any modification in, for example, feeding techniques, positioning of patients and so on. Invariably, however, the ward sister sends her trainee students. Keen to learn, these students try to put advice into practice on the ward and can be a great help. The problem is that they soon disappear to complete another aspect of their training. Thereafter no one is available to continue the programme which has been established. The remaining regular staff have not attended the workshop and therefore do not have the information necessary to carry the techniques out.

Ward sisters have their own quite legitimate reasons for allocating students to attend in-service training. Possible ones include the need to provide the students with as much relevant training as possible, shortage of trained staff available to send, lack of time, a hectic ward demanding their full attention, attending to other more pressing clinical and managerial demands and so forth.

There is no easy way round this for the therapist. Nevertheless I have found, along with colleagues from other professions, that regularity is the key to success. We have ensured that a multidisciplinary workshop on one particular topic is available on the ward at the same time on the same day every week. This is usually from 2.00–3.00 pm which covers the cross-over of the 'early' and the 'late' nursing shifts. The maximum number of staff are on duty then. Therefore there is more chance that one or two will attend. This regular slot means that, over the weeks, most staff have turned up – sometimes out of curiosity after talking to their colleagues over coffee. The regular occurrence of the workshops has resulted in word getting round. Gradually trained staff have come as well. Indeed some of the night staff have made a special, much appreciated, effort to turn up. Contact and understanding between us all has improved. Mutual respect and friendliness have grown.

Sharing nursing expertise

The in-service training available in hospital should not consist of one-way traffic from therapists to nursing staff. The nurses, too, have equally valuable expertise which could be passed onto members of other disciplines. This section describes some of the information which therapists might find useful. It is not something they are taught as part of their basic training nor when they begin work. It seems to be learnt informally in an *ad hoc*, subjective way. This means that standards of practice vary between personnel. Hence the patient's quality of care is not assured. At times his very safety may be at risk and he fails to receive a cohesive package of treatment.

The information consists of several nursing procedures which need to be common knowledge for all members of the care team. It is part of the vast store which nursing staff have at their fingertips. It reflects their expertise in a wide range of subjects. The following sections are based on my own observations. They summarize some topics in which therapists would benefit from training by nursing staff.

Reducing the risk of cross-infection

Hospitals are well-known sources of infection. Cross-infection is the transmission of infection from one person to another, or from one site on an individual to another site on the *same* person. Nosocomial infection is infection acquired by a patient from a member of staff, for example from their hands or from the equipment they are using (Clarke, 1991). There are several factors which contribute to infection. Patients are vulnerable because they have a high degree of contact with strangers and staff. Staff in addition may be carrying disease producing organisms resistant to antibiotics, for example 'methicillin-resistant staphylococcus aureus'. This organism is particularly difficult to eradicate and carries risks for patients who are immunocompromised, debilitated or with open wounds.

Obviously some therapists will have less physical contact with patients than others. Social workers, for example, may hold someone's hand to give physical comfort when interviewing them about sensitive personal details. Speech and language therapists, on the other hand, may have more invasive contact with those who have difficulty in swallowing. This may involve touching the patient inside the mouth (for example when assessing intra-oral sensation or using ice to encourage a swallow reflex) or when altering the position of the trunk and head to improve posture. Others have much greater physical contact. Occupational therapists, for example, may have skin contact with the patient when encouraging him to dress, or when helping with hygiene during toileting – physiotherapists when performing chest care or when changing the patient's position to prevent the development of contractures. This is particularly important with the unconscious brain-injured.

All these examples highlight the importance of preventing infection. Patients are particularly vulnerable because of the type of illness they have, the side-effects of drugs, and the presence of wounds or invasive procedures allowing direct entry of organisms into the body (Clarke, 1991). Clarke's advice to nursing staff should be part of the paramedical's knowledge as well. They should understand the principles of microbiology, the conditions under which microorganisms survive and multiply and the ways in which their growth may be inhibited. In addition the therapist should be familiar with the following techniques which are basic to nursing.

Hand washing

This is the simplest and most effective measure for preventing infection. However it is not used uniformly by every one. Royle and Walsh (1992) point out that the hands of hospital personnel are an important vehicle of transfer of resistant bacteria from one patient to another. They summarize some research on the subject. McFarlane (1990) demonstrated that in one study, 89% of staff failed to fully wash both hands; and Cadwaller (1989) found that not a single ward in a 600-bed district general hospital practised the hand-washing technique correctly. Phillips (1989) urges the need for washing to last 30 seconds, a quick splash under the tap is not enough.

Therapists need to have access to information about the correct procedure for handwashing. King *et al.* (1981) are a good source because they support their remarks with photographs illustrating what should be done. Important practices before and after providing care for a patient and/or handling any patient articles include the following: washing both the hands and the wrists in running water, using friction, paying attention to both dorsal and palmer surfaces and the interdigital spaces and operating the taps by the elbow rather than by the hand. None of this is taught at college.

Barrier nursing

This term describes certain medical asceptic practices used both to control the spread of and to destroy pathogenic (i.e. disease-producing) organisms (Pritchard and David, 1988). The main emphasis is on hand washing, including the use of a disinfectant such as 'Hibiscrub' and protection of clothes against bacteria. This entails the use of plastic disposable aprons, which are less permeable than cotton uniforms or clothes, and, in some cases caps, masks and footwear. Any patient who is being barrier nursed should have a sign saying 'Barrier nursing' on the door of their room.

Pritchard and David (1988) provide a useful description of the principles and practice of barrier nursing. Although theirs is a nursing textbook, it offers valuable information to the hospital therapist who, albeit unwittingly, may be a source of cross infection between patients. Indeed there is a much higher chance of this happening if she is uncertain about the rigour inherent in barrier nursing and the reasons for it. Since this is not normally part of her student training, she may have to approach a member of nursing staff on the ward for information and advice.

In my experience wards are usually busy and the senior nurse is not always available. Explanation may come from an auxiliary nurse or even the ward domestic! Their honest remarks may fail to contain vital pieces of information. This *ad hoc* method of training detracts from the patient's quality of care.

Hospital linen

Therapists in contact with patients should also familiarize themselves with ward policy for the supply and disposal of linen. Occupational therapists, for example, need to know what to do with a patient's soiled pyjamas, nightie, underwear and so forth. Speech and language therapists need to know where to find and dispose of towels and sheets used to collect secretions from the mouth.

Clean linen is usually brought to the ward each day to maintain a constant supply of each article. Dirty linen is put into bags which may be collected by the laundry porter. Nursing staff are responsible for keeping dirty linen from infectious patients separate from other linen. Therapists should also be made familiar with these procedures. For certain diseases or infections, for example, hepatitis B or AIDS, specific policies will be in force for the safe disposal of linen (Clarke, 1991).

Other important nursing expertise for the team

There spring to mind several other nursing procedures which the therapist should know. Most of these do not need to be learnt in detail. Instead a working knowledge might be sufficient; for example, what they are, why they have been done and whether they entail any special precautions when in contact with the patient. The number and type of these will depend upon where the therapist works and the illnesses she helps to treat.

Relevant issues for the hospital therapist involved might include the following: the possible effect of lifting a patient up the bed on his intravenous infusion (trapping air in the system so that it no longer functions effectively), the use of drugs regularly used for certain types of patients and their possible side-effects, nasogastric feeding, the current method of treatment for pressure sores (and any effects their own action might have on this management programme) and so on. The range of procedures can probably best be listed by the therapist herself. Nevertheless any information and training she acquires should come from a trained nurse in a systematic way – not informally and *ad hoc*.

CONCLUSION

This chapter has compared the career structure in several professions. The similarities and differences have certain implications for both staff and the patients they treat. Important points are patient consent for student intervention and basic knowledge of the career structures of other professions. Subsequent sections have highlighted aspects of student training and education which could be improved. Suggestions include more joint training of both basic theory common to the different disciplines and of practical work, in particular, joint projects and presentations. This has important implications for team work between the tutors and lecturers of different disciplines. They, too, would have to get involved with each other more closely. Contact like this might influence their awareness of the problems facing those who work in the field, unprotected by an academic environment.

In-service training, workshops and learning on the job are also discussed. There should be greater opportunities for learning alongside other professionals. Furthermore, those who run joint multidisciplinary workshops should concentrate on practical issues relevant to the audience. Content and manner of presentation are influential as well as the type of people who are participating in the workshop itself.

The final section highlights how important it is for therapists to know about some nursing procedures. Correct handwashing, barrier nursing, and other such issues are all described above. Each affects quality of care. Therefore they should be learnt according to a set standard rather than erratically, in an *ad hoc* way, practised with variability. Nurses are the important educators in these areas, just as therapists are recognized as specialists in other fields.

The diffidence of the nursing profession is reflected in the limited amount of training and education they seem to do. Therapists often run courses for nurses or are asked by senior nursing staff to talk to nursing students or show them some aspect of their work. Unfortunately the reverse is rarely true. Therapists seldom receive any training from nursing staff although it is they who have the vital expertise to share. Nor do they ask to observe an important nursing procedure. This has negative consequences. Nurses fail to realize the breadth of their expertise, often feeling inferior to the peripheral, yet specialist staff with whom they come into contact.

There is one final point to make about the suggestions above regarding training and education. It has major legal and financial implications. With the current growing emphasis on litigation in health care, training may need to be formalized. A nurse, for example, may require formal recognition, even certification, of her competence to train other staff in basic procedures. In addition she may need legal protection should anything untoward occur as a result of passing knowledge on.

Similarly formal recognition of post-qualification training may be necessary for other staff. All this costs money. Nevertheless these and similar issues have already arisen. In many health districts solicitors are working to protect the interests of their clients, who may be either patients or staff. Ongoing and potential court cases involving litigation have had implications for the professional bodies of most disciplines. Indeed most now include legal insurance as part of their membership and registration system.

In conclusion, training staff on the job is an important issue. One way of doing this might be through an extended induction programme. Many departments run these for new staff to orientate them with their surroundings and colleagues. Issues such as health and safety at work, fire safety and so forth are frequently covered. Perhaps basic issues such as hand washing and intravenous infusion should be covered in this programme. These need not involve detailed explanation. The programme should simply enable staff to recognize some techniques and to know where and whom to go to for further information.

At the same time, it is up to the individual professions to set their own standards of care. Professionals need to know when something is *not* part of their remit. In other words they need to know when they should not attempt a procedure. Issues like this are under discussion by many professional bodies and institutions. They seek to improve the quality of care by avoiding accidents and to protect their members against litigation by others.

Issues such as professional liability and certification of competence stem partly from mistakes that have happened in the past. This is not confined to health care. Examples abound in other industries where disasters and catastrophes have produced safety legislation after the event. The Chernobyl Nuclear Disaster in the Soviet Union (1986) and the Aberfan Mining Disaster in Wales (1966) are just two. Training and education in health care seems to be following a similar course. All those involved, at whatever level, may need to consider responsibility, legal protection and even certification, with guidance from their professional bodies, in-line managers and employing authorities.

7

Hospital case histories

INTRODUCTION

This chapter contains three case histories. These are drawn directly from clinical experience gained over the years while working in several hospitals in the UK. They are designed to highlight aspects of teamwork which have been raised throughout this book. There is no attempt to give an exhaustive chronological description of all aspects of each case. Only relevant medical and social details are discussed; obviously a lot more activity went on in the day-to-day management than needs to be raised here. Selected features of assessment and management have been chosen deliberately from the whole history to try to illustrate how we tried to work together in a practical way. The cases are categorized as follows:

1. Jenny – a 17-year-old head-injured victim.
2. A group of elderly patients in a long-stay hospital who suffer a range of neurological diseases as well as symptoms associated with ageing.
3. Jan – a 62-year-old Yugoslavian admitted to the local stroke unit.

CASE HISTORY 1: JENNY – HEAD-INJURED

Patient details

Jenny, aged 17, was found lying in the road at midnight. She was in a coma with no eye opening, no vocalization and no motor response. She may have been hit by a car, assaulted or have attempted suicide (as she had done in the past) but there were no witnesses. She was intubated and ventilated.

A CAT scan showed gross cerebral oedema, more evident on the right side. After 1 month at the specialist regional neurosurgical centre, she was transferred back to the District General Hospital. At that time she was unresponsive to all but painful stimuli. She opened her eyes but made no attempt to track moving objects which passed in and out of her visual field. Her limbs were hypertonic and hyperreflexic.

Joint assessment and reassessment

Jenny was seen for initial joint assessment by myself (the speech and language therapist) and the occupational therapist. Initially we used sections of the Coma Kit (Freeman, 1987) to gain a baseline measurement of her abilities. This provides a systematic means of assessing her response to certain types of stimuli. Several sections of the Kit are much easier to execute and evaluate if two people are working together. Accordingly we used a joint approach. One of us would introduce a particular stimulus (for example the sound of a whistle or a familiar odour such as mint) whilst the other recorded her response.

We continued to stimulate Jenny in this way and evaluate her response for 2–3 weeks. The physiotherapist took part in this programme as well, in addition to carrying out a programme of passive exercises designed to prevent contractures from developing further. We estalished a rota of almost twice daily sessions with two of us involved at any one time.

As Jenny's condition improved we were able to take her to the physiotherapy department. There we each took part in or observed each others assessments. The Frenchay Dysarthria Assessment (Enderby, 1988) was particularly suitable for this multidisciplinary approach. As well as assessing factors which contribute to dysarthria, for example respiratory ability and lip and laryngeal functions, this assesses the intelligibility of speech.

Jenny read aloud a selection of words and sentences presented individually on cards. The physiotherapist and the occupational therapist, who were unaware of the texts of these, actually wrote down what they thought Jenny was saying. Meanwhile I held up the stimuli for her to see. Due to the quality of her speech, the others found that they had to guess on several occasions.

Often they could not understand her at all. We were all suprised at this because, hitherto, we had believed that her speech had been improving. The exercise forced us to reconsider the influence that familiarity plays in subjective informal assessment. It led us to structure conversational activities with both the nursing staff and her family. In these the information which Jenny had to convey was totally new to her listeners. Their understanding depended upon her ability to make herself understood. This meant she had to use certain techniques taught by all three of us during her multidisciplinary therapy sessions (see below).

Joint treatment sessions

Swallowing and feeding

The physiotherapist and occupational therapist were able to move Jenny into an upright sitting position on the bedside and support her there with her head slightly flexed. Over time, they gradually reduced the amount of support they gave as her sitting balance began to improve. During these sessions, I introduced, gradually, a number of activities to facilitate her swallowing and feeding. These included various lip and tongue exercises, placing jam on her lips and coaxing her to lick it off, and introducing 2 ml of iced liquid using a syringe and kwill.

The physiotherapist, trained in the assessment and treatment of swallowing disorders, was able to evaluate the effect of this by spreading her fingers in a set pattern over Jenny's lower jaw and thyroid cartilage. This enabled her to feel whether and to what degree Jenny's tongue was moving prior to swallowing. Furthermore she could feel whether her larynx moved firstly upwards, tilting slightly outwards and then downwards during the swallow to protect her airway.

The physiotherapist's help was invaluable. In view of Jenny's posture in the early stages, it would have been physically impossible to have worked on her swallowing alone. One person could not simultaneously have supported Jenny upright, introduced liquid and monitored, by feel, the competence of her swallow reflex. Furthermore the physiotherapist kept a close eye throughout on her chest condition. Six months later Jenny was managing a semi-solid diet and fluids.

Improving sitting balance and communication

In the early stages of rehabilitation, Jenny kept her left hand fixed and extended to the side or in front of her to maintain her balance. This prevented her from using her left hand for feeding or dressing and indeed for any other useful functional activity.

We constructed, jointly, a treatment programme based on behaviour modification principles. This was aimed at altering the habit she had developed with her left hand. We wanted to discourage this and thus to improve her sitting balance. At the beginning of each 10 minute session, we positioned her hand so that it lay loosely on her lap. I then began an exercise designed to encourage Jenny to slow down her rate of speech. This involved breathing after every word. Alternatively, the occupational therapist would engage her in a right-handed writing task. These activities were designed to take up her attention for a short length of time.

At regular intervals we would pause during the activity and ask Jenny where her left hand lay. She began to notice over time that it lay loosely on her lap (rather than extended to the side or the front) and was praised for this. If she moved her left hand unconsciously during the activity, either to the side or in front of her and extended it, we simply repositioned it in the desired position on her lap.

The head-injured are known to have difficulty in concentrating and attending to several stimuli at once. Accordingly, before each session, we elected one person from the three of us to take charge of speaking. Responsibility for this function lay with the person who had engaged Jenny in the task in hand. The other two remained silent throughout, concentrating on repositioning Jenny's hand (and also trunk) when required and on keeping a score of her behaviour.

This was designed to monitor the success of our treatment approach. We counted several parameters, namely the number of times Jenny moved her hand to the 'bad' position, the times we repositioned it appropriately and the number of positive verbal reinforcements we gave. Over time Jenny abandoned the habit. Her sitting balance improved and she was able to begin using her left hand when dressing, eating and so on.

Practical Advice to Family and Ward Staff

At regular intervals the three of us wrote out, jointly, a concise, non-technical description of our aims of treatment and how staff and family could promote these. We kept the content brief and used simple, understandable headings, because we felt that nobody wanted to plough through a long professional report. They would have neither the time nor the inclination and might even be intimidated by it. Here is an example of the type of advice we gave.

Aims of treatment
1. To encourage Jenny to sit independently without using her left hand to hold onto anything.
2. To communicate intelligibly.

Activities to achieve these aims
Sitting
  (a) Do not let Jenny grip her leg with her left hand when she is sitting in her wheelchair. Encourage her to rest her left arm lightly on the arm of the wheelchair.
  (b) Encourage her to move herself around in her wheelchair using her left hand to propel the left wheel.

Speaking
  (a) If you have no idea what Jenny is saying tell her so.
  (b) Ask her to repeat the bit you have not understood but to breathe after every word she says as well.

In addition to giving all staff and the family copies of these, we pinned a copy above Jenny's bed. We also demonstrated the activities so that everybody understood what we meant and felt happy about following our suggestions.

Regular case conferences

These took place every month. Those who attended included Jenny's mother, the consultant physician in charge of her care, a member of the nursing staff from her ward, the physiotherapist, the occupational therapist, the speech and language therapist, and the social worker. Others such as the continence adviser and the clinical psychologist attended on specific occasions when necessary. Jenny's mother used the opportunity to ask specific questions and air her grievances.

The social worker provided crucial support at this stage. She made sure she had met Jenny's mother informally before each case conference and used this opportunity to go over any worries and concerns with her. She also encouraged Jenny's mother to write down both these and any questions she had. This protected her from the situation where she left the conference having forgotten to mention vital issues on the day.

By providing this support the social worker gained first-hand knowledge of fraught domestic circumstances which sometimes influenced Jenny's behaviour in hospital. She was able to pass on relevant details, with sensitivity, to the rest of us. Both the nurses on the ward and ourselves as therapists were able to allow for the effects of these. During the conference, members of the team were able to give an up-to-date report on Jenny's progress. Informal minutes were taken, typed soon afterwards and circulated to all who were involved, including the family.

CASE HISTORY 2: THE ELDERLY NEUROLOGICALLY IMPAIRED
IN A 'LONG-STAY' HOSPITAL

This section describes work with a group of elderly patients in a long-stay hospital. A more detailed account is available in Nieuwenhuis (1989). At first several factors had to be considered. These are listed below.

1. The majority of patients in the hospital were well into their seventies, eighties and nineties and suffered from illnesses associated with ageing. Diabetes, cataracts, and arthritis were compounded by features such as poor memory, confusion, incontinence, hearing loss, limited concentration span and dementia. Various long-standing neurological conditions (CVA, Parkinson's Disease) made matters even worse by producing spasticity, hemiplegia, dysphasia, dysarthria and other such symptoms.

2. The patients received no regular input from the paramedical professions. Several reasons prevented this, in particular lack of staff for the non-acute elderly wards. Another major factor was the mental and physical condition of the patients themselves. Most had received several weeks, if not

months, of rehabilitation therapy years ago immediately after their initial neurological episode. Thereafter many had suffered further neurological events which had left them severely debilitated. Any recovery had plateaued long since, hampered, in addition, by many of the ageing factors listed above. Therefore further efforts at rehabilitation were unrealistic. A more reasonable approach was to help the patients to both use and maintain their remaining skills and to work together with the nursing staff.

3. The nursing staff were, however, working at full capacity already. Their time on the wards was filled with carrying out essential nursing care (bathing, dressing, toileting and so on). They had little space or energy left to provide recreation. In addition, many of them were unaware how to stimulate and communicate with patients as debilitated as those in their care.

4. The 'Patients' Activities Department' (a centre in the hospital devoted to providing recreational pursuits) already provided many facilities for the patients, but they experienced problems in trying to carry out successfully the activities which they had devised. The staff, four trained nurses in charge of a team of volunteers, were unable to encourage participation by everyone. Many patients simply sat through the sessions, unaware of what was going on, giving no verbal or physical response. Despite Herculean efforts to reach these individuals, the staff were unable to tap the potential which they felt was there. Nevertheless they remained convinced that more could be achieved if only they could present their activities in a different way.

Up until now the Activities staff had struggled on alone valiantly. Due to a change in staffing and departmental policies, the physiotherapist and myself were able to consider how we could get involved. (Unfortunately the occupational therapy department had no one available to join us, although their staff followed our planning and activities closely.) We wanted to provide as much practical assistance as possible. This, we hoped, would assist not only the patients but also the Activities staff and the ward nursing staff.

There followed several joint informal meetings between the physiotherapist, the Activities staff and myself. We all agreed that a team approach, pooling all our resources, might produce interesting results. Some time later we had decided on several strategies. There would be group activities rather than individual treatment sessions. This would allow for the mental condition of many of the patients. None of them could concentrate for more than a few minutes at a time.

Sessions would take place both on the ward and in smaller groups in the Patients' Activities Department. Ward sessions were designed to include as many individuals as possible. They were also an attempt to involve the nursing staff without having to remove them from the ward. The small group sessions, on the other hand, provided a chance to see together patients with similar levels of ability. Ward sessions took place twice a week for about an hour. The focus of these alternated systematically. One type of session involved activities aimed at encouraging communication. I attended this one. Another type, organized by the physiotherapist, tried to encourage physical movement. The Activities staff took part in both types of session, thereby providing continuity.

The sessions in the Activities Centre occurred three times a week for about an hour and a half, and included a tea or coffee break. These involved communication and stimulation of all types. I attended every third one of these. No patient was forced to participate in the activities if they did not want to. We respected their privacy and their right to refuse.

The communication sessions involved a variety of activities. Quizzes, news reporting, card games and role play were just a few. We tried to incorporate the principles of reality orientation to reduce levels of confusion. In addition several basic practices made a vast difference to the ultimate success of reaching a patient and encouraging a response. These included using appropriate gesture to supplement speech, thereby helping those patients who had difficulty understanding what was said. Another involved alerting the patient to the fact that someone else was speaking by making hand and eye contact, calling that patient's name several times to attract his attention, and then pointing vigorously at the person, often another patient, who was speaking to him.

Other strategies entailed waiting for several seconds before conveying a message and giving a few minutes rest to someone with limited concentration span. Furthermore some patients understood the written rather than the spoken word more easily. Hence we wrote down for them many of both our own comments and those made by their neighbours in the group. We also used cards with key words and names written on them in large print to act as memory aids. We modified the surrounding environment by, for example, switching off a noisy extractor fan which distracted some patients, preventing them from attending to what was being said. Similarly we turned off background radio and television, usually sounding constantly on the ward. We moved patients from their positions around the walls into a circle. This meant that they could see each other and be aware of who was speaking to them.

The small group sessions in the Activities Centre benefitted from the introduction of certain equipment. Some patients had refused to wear their hearing aids for several years. However they accepted a specialized hand held hearing aid and speech amplifier which allowed them to hear their neighbours who had quiet voices. Some patients began to use gesture, modelled by staff, as effective ways of responding and conveying information. Above all staff became aware of their roles as listeners. This meant tolerating silences and not butting in prematurely – which often happens to avoid embarrassment during conversation. Patients were given time to respond.

The music and movement sessions, organized by the physiotherapist, proved successful as well. Activities involved, amongst others, changing position to music and passing and throwing objects to each other. Immobile and sedentary patients began to attempt to alter their position and to use their muscles by, for example, reaching their arms upwards, bending down and so forth.

Finally we organized joint communication workshops for all nursing staff in the hospital. They consisted of practical teaching sessions, using a video of the group sessions with the patients. They highlighted exactly how these severely debilitated patients could be encouraged to communicate successfully. They enabled the staff to witness exactly what the long-stay patient could achieve given a sympathetic environment and the appropriate kind of stimulation. Most of the strategies took extra time but time is precisely what the long-stay multiply impaired patient requires.

Hospital case histories

CASE HISTORY 3: JAN – CVA VICTIM

Jan was a 64-year-old retired Serbian admitted to the stroke unit of a teaching hospital with a left CVA. A subsequent CAT scan demonstrated a large left hemisphere infarct. On examination he had global dysphasia, a right homonymous hemianopia and reduced power in the right arm. However he was able to walk with the help of one person and had no swallowing problems. He was assessed by all members of the paramedical team. Both the physiotherapist and occupational therapist reported a high level of functional ability. He required only minimal guidance in walking, and in activities of daily living such as toileting, washing and dressing, grooming and bathing. His major problem was one of communication.

Both he and his wife had lived in the UK for many years, although their native language was Serbian. She spoke English well and reported that he, too, was fluent in the language prior to his stroke. A speech and language assessment in English showed that he had no understanding of what was said to him. He relied heavily on non-verbal cues such as facial expression, gesture and the context of the conversation. His wife said that he also failed to understand what was said to him in Serbian.

Her help with translation was useful in completing this basic assessment. It showed that his speech was limited to a recurrent syllable, meaningless in both languages. Furthermore his reading and writing of both were severely affected and could not be used as a means of helping communication. Severe emotional liability was a complicating factor. He spent much time in bed crying inconsolably.

The social worker had a series of informal interviews with Jan's wife and some Yugoslavian acquaintances. She established that there were various social and psychological factors at play. Although the couple had lived in the UK for decades they had little contact with anybody else. The few friends they had made belonged to the local Yugoslavian community. These people reported that the couple kept very much to themselves.

In addition Jan's wife suffered from some sort of psychosis. A persecution complex had afflicted her for many years. This was reflected in her attitude to her neighbours. She was convinced that they were conspiring against her to make her life difficult. She reported that they entered her house when she was out and began cutting up her husband's slippers. In the hospital, this persecution complex extended towards all those involved in her husband's care. She became convinced that the staff were preventing her from helping her husband to get better and became verbally abusive towards them. She also accused the nursing staff of not providing food at meal times for her husband.

She spent much of her time in tears, pacing up and down the corridor with Jan in tow. During her visits his lability increased. She was constantly doing everything for him, for example dressing him in his pyjamas, feeding him and – more importantly – talking at him in Serbian all the time. He was given no chance to try to communicate which he found difficult enough anyway due to his dysphasia. Often he simply wailed sadly throughout her long visits, calming down only after she had gone.

As speech and language therapist I could offer little help other than encouraging his wife and other staff to use non-verbal communication methods. She, however, tended to talk constantly, was unable to listen to advice or put any of it into practice. All staff on the ward began to buckle under the strain of dealing wih this complex case. Appeasing Jan's wife whilst avoiding disruptive conflict with her became a major preoccupation. We felt there was little to be done for Jan until other social and psychological factors had been tackled. However none of us felt equipped to deal with this task.

The clinical psychologist, together with the social worker, came to the rescue. They met the patient's wife on several occasions and tried to ease the situation, using their professional counselling expertise. Furthermore they contacted the couple's GP who revealed that both were well known to the practice. Indeed in the past, Jan's wife had refused repeatedly any offers of psychiatric assistance. Meanwhile on the practical side, the clinical psychologist helped to alleviate the tension on the ward. She met the patient's wife in her office nearby and acted as a sounding board. Moreover together with the social worker she met members of the local Yugoslavian community.

After several weeks, Jan's communication problems had not improved. However he no longer cried as often when his wife visited. After several multidisciplinary meetings, the consultant geriatrician in charge of his care could no longer justify keeping him in hospital. There were several reasons for this. Jan required no medical intervention and inpatient speech and language therapy was proving impossible. In addition he was by now able to care for himself and the consultant felt that the social and psychological factors, could be tackled elsewhere. Accordingly, Jan went home. He was referred for domiciliary speech and language therapy on a review basis. In addition the clinical psychologist and the social worker continued to provide domiciliary assistance and outpatient support when necessary.

The social worker discovered that the couple had planned for some years to return home to Serbia. Unfortunately all their savings were held in Jan's name. His signature would be needed to transfer the money to her before any travel arrangements could be made. After several joint sessions at their home with the community speech and language therapist, the social worker felt that Jan still did not understand the implications of signing the form. Furthermore she and the clinical psychologist felt that Jan's wife was not in a fit mental state to take control of the money. Therefore they engaged the help of the couple's solicitor. The main aim at the time of writing is to sort out the financial situation. The social worker and solicitor have contacted Jan's sister who is visiting the UK from Serbia. Political and economic turmoil in the country itself are compounding the problem. The case continues.

This case illustrates the crucial role of the social worker and the clinical psychologist. They were the people most qualified to attempt to handle the situation and its social and psychological problems. These were the very factors which prevented any rehabilitation from working. Indeed the major problem in managing the case was the mental state of Jan's wife rather than his own CVA. The social worker made a valid point when she wondered whether Jan's name at the top of medical notes should be replaced by his wife's, thus reflecting the major social and psychological factors at play.

CONCLUSION

These case histories have attempted to illustrate in practical terms how members of a health care team can work together. All three were managed in hospital although the setting was different for each one. Jenny was treated by individuals working in a district general hospital, the group of elderly patients by staff in a long-stay hospital, and Jan by those working in a city teaching hospital. In all three, certain factors had to be overcome before we could work together as a team.

Staff shortages, different caseloads and working schedules had to be sorted out. With Jenny, for example, the occupational therapist was responsible not only for the head-injured in the hospital but for other wards as well. The physiotherapist and myself, as speech and language therapist, had similar competing commitments. Furthermore we did not all work full-time in the hospital. This meant that treatment sessions and case conferences had to be arranged at a mutually suitable time. This was not always possible but we all tried to work around the problem to fit in with each other. A regular Monday morning 15-minute 'diary session' helped us to plan our week together and to cater for each others' responsibilities.

Furthermore we frequently ended up assisting with elements of each other's work. 'Non-territorial compatible personalities' (Nieuwenhuis, 1990, p. 7) proved invaluable for this. Professional jealousy would simply have been counter-productive because it would have wasted precious resources and skills (Ransome, 1990).

Similarly, in the long-stay hospital we did not start out as a formalized team. We had to take time to plan together what we thought we could achieve and modify this when we ran into problems. The nursing staff on the ward, for example, were unable to attend the ward sessions as often as we would have hoped. Accepting this and empathizing with their heavy workload was more constructive than complaining about their absence. The communication workshops, backed by ward sisters and senior nursing management, proved an effective means of getting round the problem.

Working together in all three cases had several advantages. It encouraged those involved to place the patient and his family at the centre of their activities. This led to a more coordinated service, focusing on the needs at the time rather than on individual professional roles. No one person in the team had all the answers in dealing with any of the cases. This meant that any success would lie in combining skills and tackling areas of overlap constructively. This reduced the chances of interprofessional jealousies creating barriers between the different members of staff (Squires and Taylor, 1988).

Other benefits included learning about each other's areas of expertise. In Jenny's case I learnt about various physiotherapy and occupational therapy assessment procedures and also about their treatment techniques. Similarly, with the group of elderly patients the physiotherapist and myself witnessed at first hand the dedication shown by staff involved in caring for the long-stay elderly patient who is multiply impaired. The Patients' Activities staff were particularly impressive in this respect. They carried on working with these patients long after the rehabilitation therapists had withdrawn. Often they received no feedback or reinforcement of any kind which was soul-destroying. They, in turn, appreciated the chance to share our expertise. We all gained from the experience because we supported and encouraged each other, pooling our knowledge and resources. This is very important for effective teamwork.

'Part of an employee's enjoyment of her job is the professional stroking she gets from colleagues and the fact that she likes the people she is around' (Hamdy *et al.*, 1990, p. 136). Pooling of knowledge like this often resulted in a rejuvenated, innovative approach from all concerned. For example, with Jenny, when one activity was not working as hoped, one of us would suggest an alternative way of presenting it. Often this made a crucial difference. It also made us think more objectively about our treatment approach. In Jan's case following joint discussion with the social worker and the clinical psychologist, we all concluded that treatment of speech and language was not the main priority – especially because of the social and psychological factors at play. Handling his domestic circumstances was more important at this stage because these affected his mood and well-being. My colleagues were much more qualified to deal with this than I was. However I maintained regular contact with them – both to learn how they were getting on with the case and to advise about communication if necessary.

Another practical benefit of working together involved the joint writing of reports. In Jenny's case, joint professional reports, both for the medical notes and for her mother and the ward staff, prompted us to use understandable terms, clear to all. We limited the use of obscure technical jargon. This practice arose partly because we found initially that we even questioned each other's terms, not understanding them fully. We conjectured that if this was the case amongst three people supposedly familiar with each other's work, it would be even worse for those not directly involved. This practice also reduced unnecessary paperwork. A byproduct of our improved communication was a high degree of job satisfaction. Unfortunately the hospital did not use the POMR system (see Chapter 4) which might have helped even further.

8

Community case histories

This chapter is devoted to describing certain aspects of teamwork in the community. It is based directly on personal experience and consists of four sections (including two case histories)
subdivided in the following way.

1. Case history 1 – David, a 64-year-old suffering from motor
   neurone disease.
2. Case history 2 – Adam, a 25-year-old who sustained a
   severe head injury.
3. An informal investigation into teamwork at two locations
   in the community.
4. Conclusion.

The case histories, as in Chapter 7, do not include a full
description of all the details. Only relevant factors highlighting
points of particular interest are discussed. The two cases,
together with the informal investigation, reflect the efforts of
various individuals to work together outside a hospital context.

CASE HISTORY 1

David was a 64-year-old retired factory worker who lived at
home with his wife. He had two married sons, one of whom
lived locally. The other lived about 2 hours drive away. He had
three grandchildren. David's case came to light when his GP
referred him to the speech and language therapist for help with
communication. The initial referral letter reported that he had
Alzheimer's disease and unintelligible speech. His previous
medical history was unremarkable.

History and symptoms

Soon after receiving the referral, I met David and his wife at
home for the first time. He was able to walk independently and
reported that he required no help with daily activities such
as dressing, bathing and toileting. He obviously understood

without difficulty everything that was said to him. His speech, however, was limited to continuous voicing marked by crude distinctions in vowel quality. There were no recognizeable consonant sounds and he relied on writing to communicate. The content of this was appropriate, fully grammatical and contained no spelling errors.

His house was full of used bits of paper containing messages to his wife and family. He kept a large notebook close by, alert to any conversation directed towards him and ready to scribble answers down as quickly as possible. His written messages showed none of the disordered thought processes associated with Alzheimer's disease.

In addition he dribbled constantly. His wife reported that he also coughed repeatedly when drinking tea or coffee and occasionally had problems in eating and swallowing particular types of food. I observed all these features during this first visit. The problems with his speech, he claimed, had developed gradually over the past few months, the swallowing difficulties in the last few weeks.

Verifying the diagnosis

Following a diagnosis of Alzheimer's disease from the GP, David's wife had contacted the Alzheimer's Disease Society for further information. They sent her various pamphlets and newsheets which described the nature of the conditon, its expected course and how best to manage the situation at home. She said, however, that she did not think her husband showed the symptoms highlighted in the literature. He, too, had formed the same opinion, having read the facts himself.

At this stage, I also questioned the diagnosis of Alzheimer's disease. David's history and presentation suggested some other progressive degenerative neurological condition affecting the bulbar musculature. Fasciculation of the tongue and wasting of muscles of the neck pointed to motor neurone disease. Obviously the treatment and management for this would be completely different to that for Alzheimer's disease (see Chapter 1). The first priority, therefore, was a referral to a neurologist who would be able to verify the diagnosis.

The GP, approached by telephone, was reluctant to do this for reasons of his own. Accordingly I spoke to the community physiotherapist whose help and support proved invaluable. She visited David at home and immediately suspected motor neurone disease in view of his history and further signs of muscle wasting and weakness which she observed in his hands. She agreed with the need for an immediate specialist neurological opinion.

Together we approached informally, face-to-face, a consultant physician at the local district hospital. We outlined the case and the management problems facing us. He contrived, by diplomatic means of his own, to admit David to hospital. There he was seen immediately by the consultant neurologist who diagnosed motor neurone disease and broke the news to his wife. She was devastated and asked the consultant not to tell her husband until she had come to terms with the diagnosis herself over the next few days.

Brief hospital intervention

While in hospital David also underwent full assessment from the hospital paramedical team. He needed little direct practical assistance from occupational therapy at this stage. The physiotherapist, however, monitored his chest condition closely and the speech and language therapist felt that his swallowing problems were severe enough for him to be at constant risk of aspiration. He coughed and choked uncontrollably for long periods, both on his own saliva and on small amounts of liquids and food of all consistencies. The consultant agreed to stop all oral intake of food and drink in the interests of safety. He insisted upon some sort of alternative feeding regime.

Accordingly the hospital dietician met David and arranged permanent long-term nasogastric feeding, tailored to his nutritional requirements (feeding by long-term percutaneous endoscopic gastrostomy was not yet an option at this particular hospital). In addition the speech and language therapy department tackled the problem of his communication. Writing was proving to be rather laborious, particularly for the person waiting for him to complete his text. A 'Lightwriter' (see Chapter 4) offered him a means of conveying messages more quickly than pen and paper alone. Nevertheless, on the whole, he continued to prefer writing because he felt more in control of his situation. He developed a system whereby he used the 'Lightwriter' with certain staff members on the ward but used writing with his family.

Community support

David went home after 3 days. The consultant had told him that he did not have Alzheimer's disease, as diagnosed by his GP, but 'some other neurological condition'. David himself actually believed he had suffered a stroke. He was delighted to realize that he was not suffering from progressive dementia as originally thought. He did not question the consultant further at this stage. When he was discharged, the hospital team transferred his case to a number of community professionals for continued support at home. These included the dietician, physiotherapist, speech and language therapist, the district nurse, and a Macmillan nurse, trained to deal with terminal illness and its emotional and psychological consequences. The community dietician continued to monitor David's weight, modifying his nasogastric feeds as appropriate. She saw him at home on a review basis every 2 weeks or so. The district nurse dealt with the practicalities of giving these feeds, showing his wife what to do and helping her to manage any problems which arose.

Over the next few weeks David's condition began to deteriorate. He was finding it progressively more difficult to stay upright, whilst both sitting and standing, due to muscle fatigue. His head was beginning to drop and his back was becoming hunched. The community physiotherapist became directly involved. She helped David and his wife to deal with the problem of the altered posture of his trunk and limbs.

She gave practical advice, demonstrating what could be done. To help minimize the effect of gravity on his body, she reclined him back from the vertical both when he was sitting in his armchair and when he was lying in bed. Furthermore she showed them how to support the weight of his arms with bean-bag cushions. This relieved the pain and discomfort in his neck. Finally she helped with the problem of his joints which were beginning to get stiff and painful. They needed to be moved regularly to prevent contractures from developing. She explained what was wrong and taught his wife what to do to help. Among other tasks my involvement as community speech and language therapist lay in monitoring the effectiveness of his communication and offering advice and assistance when necessary.

Telling the patient the diagnosis

Despite all this work, one major factor hampered our management of this case – namely David's ignorance of the nature of his illness and its prognosis. Both his wife and his sons insisted that we did not tell him until they felt ready to handle the situation. We were all uneasy about this, and felt David deserved honesty from everyone. However we were in a difficult position because the medical team had respected the family's wishes so far.

We arranged a team meeting to discuss the matter further. Unfortunately neither the GP nor the consultant neurologist were able to attend. During the meeting, we all recognized the need for someone to tell David his diagnosis. We agreed that the Macmillan nurse, with specialist expertise in counselling, was the best equipped to handle this task. However she was reluctant to antagonize David's wife, who was already under a great deal of emotional stress. We all decided that, in the circumstances, the diagnosis should really be given by the consultant neurologist. The Macmillan nurse would then be able to support both partners as the need arose.

Meanwhile David's continued ignorance about the truth, together with his wife's behaviour, made our management of the case increasingly difficult. Anyone from the team who visited the couple faced a tense situation. David would note the person's arrival from the living room, where he spent most of his time. Meanwhile his wife would intercept the visitor at the door and have a hurried whispered conversation about her husband's deteriorating condition, often ending up in tears. Thereafter she would usher the visitor in to see him, disappearing into the kitchen until she had composed herself.

David would make occasional remarks, via his 'Lightwriter' or in writing, about his lack of progress. However he never asked outright what he suffered from. His wife would then reappear, to give comments such as 'He looks a lot better, doesn't he?' appealing to the visitor for verification. In effect she was asking us to collude in her husband's deception, possibly because this was the only way she could handle the situation herself. Despite the difficulties, we did not lie about any imaginary improvements but gave honest opinions about his condition on the days we visited.

I contacted the consultant neurologist and explained the delicate nature of the situation. He arranged to see the couple together with a view to telling David the diagnosis. The Macmillan nurse was ready to meet the couple immediately after this interview to provide support. However David's wife spoke privately to the consultant just before the appointment and asked him again not to let her husband know his diagnosis and its implications. For whatever reasons, he respected her wishes. He examined David, agreed that he had not improved but still did not tell him what was wrong. The couple returned home and the situation remained unsolved. David continued to assume he had suffered a stroke.

Two days later he was admitted to hospital with severe breathlessness and a sudden deterioration in his condition. Fortunately the drugs diamorphine, chlorpromazine and hyoscine relieved his distress. These continued over the next few days by subcutaneous infusion and he died peacefully with his wife and sons by his bedside.

Problems highlighted by the case

Unfortunately, despite our diplomatic efforts, David never discovered the truth about his illness. This had practical and emotional consequences. He never had the chance to wind up his affairs or discuss matters with his wife and family. Understandably she now felt not only grief but guilt at her conduct before his death. She met the Macmillan nurse several times for support and counselling and suffered from severe depression for some time.

Several factors were relevant for the professionals in handling this case. The Macmillan nurse discovered, early on, that David and his wife felt bombarded by the number of people who were visiting. Accordingly she assumed, by common consent, the role of key worker to coordinate the visits of the other staff. This allowed us to space our visits out and to offer our various types of help and support when it was most needed. The case also highlighted that teamwork does not necessarily guarantee a satisfactory outcome. Obviously, David should have known the truth about his diagnosis and been allowed to face it with support and help. Deception is no help to anyone, particularly the adult neurologically impaired. We all felt a professional loyalty to David as the patient. In addition we all sympathized with his wife and recognized the strain she was under. In the long-run, however, our team efforts to cater for both husband and wife proved unsuccessful.

Care of the dying frequently involves handling both the patient's and the relatives' knowledge or ignorance of the diagnosis. Nursing texts advocate adopting a sympathetic, supportive attitude but leaving the doctor to answer any questions directly (Clarke, 1991). Unfortunately, however, a doctor's training seldom guides him how to respond. Baldwin and Hopcroft (1987), both housemen themselves, advise their peers to tell the patient his diagnosis and prognosis in the following way. 'In our experience, it is best to let the patient lead the way in discussion of diagnosis and prognosis. Withhold information until the patient indicates that he is prepared to know, then gradually tell him.' (p. 48) Unfortunately this strategy was no help to the rest of the team in David's case and reflects the non-holistic approach of medicine. Baldwin and Hopcroft do admit later, however, that maintaining relatives' fragile conspiracies is unhelpful – 'informed discussion with all concerned parties is the key to honesty in the management of the terminally ill'. (p. 48). Our difficulty lay in trying to bring this about.

We believed as a team that review by the consultant neurologist, with an honest explanation of the diagnosis, was the best way of handling the situation at the time. Our efforts foundered because the consultant thought differently. The case closed in an unsatisfactory way leaving us wondering whether we should have acted differently from the outset. It highlights how the best intentioned plans may go awry, despite the united efforts of several team members.

CASE HISTORY 2

Adam was a 25-year-old who had suffered a severe head injury in France following a road traffic accident 4 years earlier. He had recently moved into the area with his mother. He lay in a persistent vegetative state at home. He was able to open his eyes but did not appear to focus on anything within his visual field. All four limbs showed marked spasticity and he made no voluntary movement. His swallowing reflex was impaired although he was able to take, from his mother, small amounts of both fluid and a semi-solid diet. Chewing and swallowing were laboriously slow. Overnight feeding by a percutaneous endoscopic gastrostomy supplemented his oral intake. His communication was non-existent. He showed no sign of understanding anything, either spoken or written. He occasionally grunted but otherwise produced no speech.

Adam's mother looked after him with some community support. The district nurse visited once a day and a local voluntary group provided further help. They came to sit with him to allow her to go out, arranging their visits on a systematic rota. Adam's mother had campaigned widely for funds to help him and had succeeded in buying a specially equipped car to take him out, although she had not yet passed her driving test.

The community physiotherapist had been involved with Adam for some weeks. She visited him on a review basis to monitor his chest condition and to provide advice and assistance on handling and positioning. Passive exercises helped to prevent further development of contractures. She referred Adam to me because his mother had reported that he was starting to speak.

I met Adam at home and found his condition no different from that reported above. He showed no response when I played his stereo loudly, alternately, beside both ears. He did not respond to his name or to touch. He failed to track anything which passed across his visual field. He showed no sign of understanding and made no attempt to communicate. His mother reported, however, that he said two to three word sentences when I was not around. At the same time, she told the physiotherapist that he was moving his hands and legs when she asked him to.

We both made several weekly to fortnightly visits over the next few weeks. We also liaised with the district nurse and the local voluntary group. There was no change in Adam's condition during any of our visits. His mother, however became increasingly hostile. She insisted repeatedly that he was talking and moving, activities which seemed impossible given his persistent vegetative state. Over time the physiotherapist and I both concluded that she was deluding herself as a means of survival.

Adam's case highlights the situation which the community professional may encounter. She may face relatives who are desperate to see improvement in their loved one or else despair altogether. Recovery has plateaued and the patient is severely disabled – yet the family need to have some hope to hang onto. In this situation, stating the professional truth while empathizing with the family create difficult problems. These are particularly hard to handle when the patient's condition and lack of progress for several years suggest that further regular input is inappropriate.

We both stated, as sensitively as possible, that Adam's condition was static. We said, moreover, that improvement at this late stage and after such severe injuries was unexpected. In addition we contacted Adam's GP to discuss the situation: he was unable to offer further assistance, saying that Adam's mother confronted all health care staff with the same uncorroborated claims.

Moreover she had refused help from both a social worker and a clinical psychologist who might have been able to help her face the truth, using their professional counselling expertise. We considered enlisting the help of Headway, the national association concerned with helping the head-injured and their carers (see Chapter 2). This avenue, too, proved unfruitful. We discovered that Adam's mother was already an active member of the local group. Indeed other members reported that she tended to dominate meetings with lengthy accounts of Adam's apparent progress.

All our efforts to help her to face the truth of the situation were to no avail. Nevertheless we kept Adam under review for some weeks because she still wanted our involvement (and because we wanted to ensure beyond doubt that her accounts of his behaviour were indeed fantasy). Eventually after several weeks, for whatever reason, her hostility waned. She seemed to be content with our intermittent visits and no longer reported improvements such as those reported above. We were both able to reduce our visits to monthly and then 3-monthly review. She was quite amicable about this. Adam's condition remained unchanged throughout this time. Finally after several months Adam's mother stated that she did not wish any further visits at present. She agreed to contact us again should she need further advice or review.

This case illustrates the central role of the patient's relative which affects the work of the team. Adam's mother's attitude influenced not only what we both did but also the pace of events. We had to respect her reluctance to accept any psychological help, even though this made the situation more difficult to handle. Her pretence and self-delusion were her means of survival. They were as important in our teamwork as our assessment and management of Adam's condition.

THE 'PATCH SYSTEM' AND PRIMARY HEALTH CARE TEAMS

In the UK, the importance of teamwork in the community features in several significant NHS reports. There is a general acceptance that it improves the services available to patients.

It enables them to call on a wider range of skills than any one individual may have. Teamwork also provides the team with an opportunity to support itself by discussing difficult personalities and by sharing the burden of responsibility and care.

Jarman, 1988, p. 88

Following Cumberledge (1986) and subsequent reports, the 'patch system' developed in many health districts. This is a community-based health care delivery system. Different professionals within a specific area or 'patch' are responsible for the health care of the resident population. Patch boundaries are determined by factors such as the location of GP practices and the areas covered by the Department of Social Services. Several patches have a **primary health care team**. This consists of a group of professionals who work together to provide health care outside a hospital setting. Some primary health care teams are linked to their local community hospital, often served by the local GPs. This allows continuity of care.

Some teams have a manager responsible for district nurses, health visitors, school nurses, family planning nurses and clinic activities. His role includes assessing local health needs, setting priorities, managing a budget, recruiting staff, liaising with other departments, ensuring good communications, assessing team needs, improving teamwork and monitoring activity. In larger health care teams, this person is a full-time manager. In the smaller teams, he may also have a clinical commitment in, for example, nursing, physiotherapy and so forth.

There follows a description of an informal research project into some aspects of community team care. This investigated, by a series of informal interviews, the degree of teamwork and attitudes to it at two contrasting locations:

1. An urban GP practice with an existing primary health care team.
2. A rural 'patch' isolated from major towns and centres. This did not yet operate fully and did not have a patch manager.

Seven different community professions were interviewed:

• GPs
• District nurses
• Health visitors
• Community psychiatric nurses
• Community physiotherapists
• Community occupational therapists
• Community speech and language therapists

Nieuwenhuis (1988–1989) gives a full account of the project, including the reasons behind the choice of subject and the method of data collection. The following description summarizes those points relevant to teamwork in the community.

The primary health care team in an urban GP practice

This team was formed several years ago in an effort to improve fact-to-face contact between staff based at the practice. For the first 2 years meetings took place every 2–3 months. These were attended by nursing staff and, intermittently, by GPs depending upon their available time and commitment to the team. Informal *ad hoc* discussion arose about individual patients, information was exchanged and problems aired.

In recent years, meetings took place more often. Their format gradually altered and additional staff attended. Rather than discussing patients, team members chose to investigate specific pre-set topics. These were wide and varied. Accordingly some individuals found them to be more relevant to their daily work than others. However everyone said they generated interesting ideas. Different topics for discussion included the following areas:

- The safe disposal of drugs.
- The chairmanship of the team (now rotated amongst the practice nurses).
- The community alcohol abuse and drug service.
- Measles, mumps and rubella immunization.
- Presentations by an occupational therapist and the health authority's legal adviser.
- Domiciliary physiotherapy cover.
- The Macmillan nurse scheme.
- Neighbourhood nursing.

Successful primary health care team meetings

Staff considered the meetings to be successful for many reasons. Firstly the team had a democratic outlook. No individual acted as overall leader or manager. Instead a chairman, elected each year, organized and coordinated each meeting according to an agreed agenda. Moreover regular invitations to specific guest speakers ensured that the time spent was both interesting and worthwhile. A secretary who took and circulated the minutes of each meeting prompted good communication between the team members. Most importantly a free sandwich lunch, provided by the GPs, and a permanent venue (a room in the practice) encouraged people to attend.

The rural 'patch'

This had been formed by a management team from the local health authority. It covered a large geographical area and included several GPs' practices, although the doctors from these had little contact with each other, and, in some cases, none at all. Most community staff within the 'patch' worked in isolation, meeting rarely and often by chance at the different GPs' surgeries or even at a patient's home. They had no headquarters or recognized leader and were linked only by their presence within boundaries of the geographical area proposed by the health authority team.

Reasons preventing closer teamwork at both locations

Staff in the urban practice listed various features which prevented them from working together more closely. Firstly face-
to-face contact at team meetings varied according to personal
inclination and available time. Regular attenders included some
GPs, the district nurses, health visitors and the community
physiotherapist. Other staff were less committed. This included
the remaining GPs from the practice, two community psychiatric nurses, the occupational therapist and the community
speech and language therapist. These nurses and therapists
rarely turned up because they had allegiances and responsibilities to other surgeries and professional groups. Moreover,
they shared their caseloads with other colleagues.

Other reasons preventing closer teamwork were common to
both locations. In both the rural 'patch' and the urban practice,
the interviews highlighted a lack of awareness about each
others' professions and responsibilities. One person often
assumed that another was unwilling to liaise with them – mainly
because the two parties never had any contact. Lack of understanding like this led to ill-feeling and hostility. Frequent
remarks like 'Oh, they don't want anything to do with us' and
'we've never seen "X" here ever!' illustrate this attitude.

In addition, practical issues hampered closer teamwork. Staff
reported that they had little contact with those who were not
based at or who did not visit their premises as part of their
working routine. Basic difficulties were, for example, the distance people had to travel and the time they had available. The
enthusiasm for teamwork also appeared to be linked with a
person's age or employment status. Members of staff nearing
retirement and some part-time workers were less willing to alter
their working practices to cater for team meetings. Conversely,
most younger members of staff and those working full-time
were prepared to change their routine if necessary.

Nearly everyone, including the GPs had a basic knowledge
of the services offered by others, but many felt that their own
roles were misunderstood by both other staff and the general
public. 'Nobody really knows what I do' was a common complaint. In the rural patch, the possibility of introducing a patch
manager was particularly controversial. Most staff wanted to
see a non-managerial coordinator with secretarial or adminis-

trative ability who could act as a link between individuals when necessary. They viewed a more senior qualified manager as a threat to their own positions and professional autonomy.

Discussion

This informal study produced several conclusions. Some of these are relevant for any junior 'grass-roots' professional working in the community and also for their managers. Firstly, separation by location and distance were major factors contributing to poor liaison between staff. This created little opportunity for face-to-face contact (judged by most interviewees to be highly important in establishing and maintaining good relations). Poor communication led to lack of understanding between professionals about each others' roles, areas of expertise, professional structure and geographical areas of responsibility. Finally the success of teamwork was influenced by the age and employment status of individual professionals.

The study also had several implications for anyone trying to build a team in the community. Results suggest that existing levels of communication and liaison between professionals need to improve *before* teams are formed. There is no point in trying to impose a system, top down, from management to junior staff. This will have little chance of success and would only antagonize the junior staff, creating friction and conflict. Instead, all staff who will be affected by a team should be consulted and involved in some way in the planning process.

There are practical ways of achieving this. Staff could be encouraged to prepare an informal summary of their contact location, professional role, place within their organizational structure and their possible level of involvement with other professionals. A series of meetings over time might help to devolve this information to all those who would be involved in the team. Each profession could give a short 20-minute presentation of the main points of their summary. Thereafter, collating the information together in a team booklet would provide a useful source of general information. This would be a valuable written aid to spreading communication. It would also be useful for any new team members who join later on.

Plans like this entail strenuous attempts at practical organization. Obviously somebody, acceptable to all, needs to take on the task. Nevertheless such efforts might bear fruit in the long term by gaining everyone's support and cooperation. This is vital for any community team, where individuals need to coordinate their activities.

CONCLUSION

This chapter has looked at two case histories and an informal study of teamwork at two community locations. Several conclusions can be drawn. Firstly developing and maintaining a team in the community is more difficult than doing the same thing in hospital. Practical factors hamper the operations of the community team (for example lack of opportunity for contact, responsibility for a wide geographical location, the time taken to travel to patients' homes and to administrative meetings, lack of access to one set of notes and so forth).

Barber and Kratz (1980) describe the difficulties of using the team approach in the community as compared to that used in a hospital. Within the community each profession has long been accustomed to professional autonomy. Each has developed an identity that has permitted independent decision-making and each has assumed professional responsibility. The individual disciplines do not have access to the structure inherent in hospital work. Indeed the staffing of a hospital is based strictly on a hierarchical system with each individual discipline and department and within the totality of the parts that make up the whole. The senior consultant is at the top. Decision making stems from the medical profession. In the community, on the other hand, teamwork means that each profession needs to find its own identity in the team and develop an approach to working together.

Secondly, the case histories illustrate how family involvement has a major influence on managing any case in the community. This probably occurs because events actually take place in the home and because the family dictate the pace of events. Often community health workers have to deal with the emotional and psycho-social pressures of the family as much as they have to treat the patient. Indeed managing the family may become equally as important as seeing the patient because family are the very people on whom care at home eventually depends. They are the crucial members of the health care team.

Hospital workers, on the other hand, can rely on the hospital as the main carer. This difference can make the job slightly easier in some instances. It is more predictable and familiar and does not have the emotional problems of the home environment. It also allows more opportunity for contact between team members because everything happens on one site rather than scattered between different homes in the community. Issues relevant to community and hospital work are discussed further in the final chapter of this book.

9

Conclusion

The concept of teamwork within health care is not new. Indeed team care in medicine is the subject of a large number of texts and articles, spanning many years. Most of these agree that the team approach enhances overall patient care. Various issues, which recur in the literature, are said to contribute to successful team dynamics (Barber and Kratz, 1980; Fussey and Giles, 1988; Squires, 1988; Garner, 1990; Smyth, 1990). They include the need to blurr professional roles, restrict professional isolation, abandon territorial behaviour, reduce inter-departmental jealousies, and avoid any misunderstanding and misperception of each others' roles. There is further emphasis in some texts on altering tradition, training and education. This is considered a way of encouraging people to work together, thereby helping to meet the needs of the patient and his family.

DISCUSSION

The discussion in previous chapters allows various conclusions and recommendations to be drawn. These may be of interest to students of different disciplines, their tutors and lecturers, and professionals working in different jobs. They will be discussed below.

Administrative and bureaucratic issues

Many staff taking up a new post may find references to teamwork in their job descriptions. Phrases indicating this include examples such as 'liaison with staff members from other disciplines', 'participation in teamwork' and 'coordination of the service with other specialities across the district'. These reflect an attempt by managers to encourage their staff to link up with other individuals. They imply that a certain amount of teamwork should take place. Without them, the new recruit might end up working primarily on her own in varying degrees of isolation.

Nevertheless additional comments in the job description might improve the chances of 'liaison', 'participation', and 'coordination'. Perhaps job descriptions should contain specific information on the type and nature of teamwork expected in the post (cf. Edwards and Hanley, 1989, p. 375). This would involve spelling out exactly who should be approached and for what reason. A speech and language therapist, for example, may be responsible for the assessment, treatment and management of dysphagia as part of her work. Perhaps her job description should contain recommendations such as 'liaison with the physiotherapist and nursing staff with regard to posture and chest condition', 'contact with the occupational therapist for appropriate seating and feeding equipment', and so on.

Written detail like this would have some advantages: it would clarify for the individual exactly what she should be doing; in other words, who she should contact and for what reason. It would let her know what the other person was responsible for and why she should approach them. In addition the more specific job description would clarify the roles of the other disciplines, thereby limiting opportunities for misunderstanding and misperception. These often result in hostility and breakdown in communication (see Chapter 3).

Nevertheless job descriptions like this carry certain disadvantages. Firstly, they would be longer because specifying individual actions would take up more room on the page. This exercise might be regarded as both time consuming and wasteful. An alternative would be to include the information in each profession's 'departmental policy' (see Chapter 6) and ensure that it is both accessed by the new recruit and put into practice.

There is a second disadvantage to specifying teamwork within an individual's job description. It would involve more thought from those managers and personnel departments who are involved in recruiting new staff. Extra work imposed is never a popular move. Perhaps, however, the information could be included in the manager's specific guidelines to staff about their responsibilities and when and where further expertise should be sought. There is a final drawback to specifying in job descriptions the exact nature of teamwork expected. This is the professional vulnerability which it might entail. In other words, it could weaken the individual's legal protection. Stating that an action should take place entails that the professional should make every effort to perform it. If she fails to meet the required standard, legal action and complaints might ensue. Drawbacks such as these would have to be weighed against the benefits for enhanced teamwork which might ensure better patient care.

Detailed written specification of action is relevant to other areas besides job descriptions. It can be useful when giving instructions to other staff or when recording a patient's progress. Ideally, as discussed in Chapter 4, a uniform set of patient notes should exist. These should be accessible to all staff. In reality, however, most community and hospital workers continue to keep their own professional notes. Indeed few of us have the managerial clout or opportunity to alter the existing system and simply have to get on with the job as best as we can.

Accordingly, writing in (for example) the nursing Kardex and care plan (see Chapter 4) may be the only means of conveying information to the nursing staff. Since they provide continuity of care, spelling out instructions in detail can be vital. This could include an indication of the amount of time needed to do something. The speech and language therapist, for example, might specify the amount of time to be spent communicating with the patient in a particular way (cf. Cole, 1986). Similarly, the physiotherapist might specify at what time and in what way a patient should be repositioned and so on.

Such recommendations, nevertheless, would require major liaison between senior nursing staff and the other professions. Therapists would need to appreciate the demands already made upon a nurse's time and to allow for these in their recommendations. Ward sisters would need to perceive the importance of carrying out the therapists' instructions. Despite these drawbacks, the suggestion is not totally ludicrous, especially in the light of attempts by nurses to evaluate their actions. Some hospitals in the UK have tried to itemize each nursing action in terms of the time it takes to perform it. Collating information like this allows senior nursing staff on the ward to evaluate their manpower needs and thus estimate how many nurses they need for how many patients.

Problems, of course, do arise – just as they do with other types of nursing system such as primary nursing (see Chapter 5). What happens, for example, when a nurse is moved to another ward to make up for a shortage of staff elsewhere? And what about the unplanned emergencies which frequently arise? Nevertheless by beginning to measure how long it takes to carry out their instructions, therapists may improve communication and understanding with their nursing colleagues.

Managers have a vital role to play. Their input is crucial if liaison on this scale is to work. They need to ensure that their staff know about the record keeping of other professions. They also need to direct them how to contribute to these in a readable, accessible way, using a minimum of jargon. It is extremely important to know the intended audience and their needs as far as your own profession is involved. Enlightened managers are those who offer their staff informative advice about the other professions. This encourages earlier recognition and rigorous use of the systems already in operation. Such action would prevent, for example, the newly qualified therapist writing her reports in the medical notes, only to discover months later, that they were not consulted by the nursing staff whom she wished to address.

This assumes that managers, too, learn more about their fellow health care professions, namely how they write their reports and how to add efficiently and succinctly to these if necessary. In the ideal world, a common system would exist, avoiding the need to consult and duplicate notes in different sources. Unfortunately practices in health care are not ideal, particularly for those well down the managerial line. They simply have to operate within an existing system, often frustratingly restrictive and labour intensive.

A second administrative and bureaucratic issue arises from the preceding chapters. This concerns the formalities of organization and planning necessary to start a working team. In some cases, teamwork is preceded by meetings amongst members of staff from various disciplines. These are used to set forth aims and objectives and establish procedures (for example referral procedure, discharge procedure, report writing and so on). Naturally these issues are very important. They dictate the way in which members of the team are supposed to work together. Nevertheless an informal approach can work well too. This less structured situation arose in several of the cases described in Chapters 7 and 8.

Teamwork prospered when people from different disciplines simply shared their thoughts about individual cases during informal encounters (for example during a social visit to the occupational therapy department). This led to informal joint sessions with the patient which, in turn, generated further ideas and treatment techniques. Our expertise grew as we became more accustomed to working with each other and picking each others' brains.

Successful teamwork does not, therefore, necessarily rely on formal rules and structures. Indeed we had none of these to refer to. We simply tried to work together with each other as the situation arose. Perhaps, in some cases, formal procedures can be listed *after* people have had some experience of trying to work together. This allows the policy to be based directly on common practical experiences, taking account of successes and failures. It probably works best where only a small number of people are involved, where contact is easy and where the individuals get on with each other anyway.

And what about the self-help groups themselves? The preceding chapters – particularly Chapter 2 – illustrate their influence in promoting teamwork. This is reflected in the different range of professionals from whom they have succeeded in gaining support. Indeed many disciplines now contribute to aspects of the self-help group literature, their information combining to offer a joint package for patients and their families. The Motor Neurone Disease Association and The Multiple Sclerosis Society of Great Britain and Northern Ireland even have pamphlets aimed at the professionals themselves.

This influence on teamwork is not restricted to self-help groups for the adult with acquired neurological brain damage. It arises in other fields where groups have formed in direct response to the needs of the patient. 'Changing Faces', for example, was launched in May 1992. It is a charity which aims to give practical and psychological help to those with facial disfigurement. It advertises teamwork because it has enlisted the support of plastic surgeons and psychologists.

This influence on promoting teamwork could be strengthened

by closer contact between the self-help groups themselves. Unfortunately, at present, they tend to work in isolation. Competition for government and public interest and funding may be one of the reasons. Whatever the cause, it can contribute to ill-feeling between groups who are campaigning for the needs of their members. An example appeared in the November 1990 issue of the Alzheimer's Disease Society Newsletter. A review of a book entitled 'Working Alongside Carers' (Sutcliff, 1990) asked why the Society was not mentioned with other organizations that support carers or give specialist information. One possible solution to avert situations like this could be joint advertising and lobbying by the self-help groups on certain issues (such as teamwork). Beneficial spin-offs would include a higher profile for the groups themselves and access to a wider range of common information.

Fortunately there is an optimistic outlook for this approach. The Motor Neurone Disease Association is helping to fund a new approach for the care and support of people with motor neurone disease, Parkinson's disease, multiple sclerosis, dystonia and ataxia. Already piloted on patients with Parkinson's disease, both they and staff have found it is a helpful way to work. A 'neuro-care team' at the Harold Wood hospital, Romford, Essex, straddles the hospital/community divide, recognizes patients as a whole, responds to their needs and involves them and their carers in monitoring and decision making. It aims to provide a co-ordinated, flexible, high quality service. This is delivered to patients who face the prospect of increasing disability from neurological illnesses. They also have to confront the uncertainty which stems from no available cure at present and no clear pattern of progression for their disease (Motor Neurone Disease Association Newsletter, Spring 1990: pp. 11–12; Oxtoby, 1990).

Practical issues

The preceding chapters also give rise to several practical suggestions. These, too, may be of interest to students, qualified staff and professional managers both in hospitals and in the community. Firstly, any team work will be influenced by the environment in which its members have to work. I have worked in various locations in hospitals and in the community and have noticed some common patterns. Generally speaking, old premises make teamwork more difficult. The environment seems to affect the attitudes, motivation and performance of the staff involved. This is particularly true in those hospitals for infectious diseases such as tuberculosis. Despite regular maintenance, the previous history of the place seems to permeate the very walls and affect the people therein.

This process applies to patients as well as staff. Local people, especially the elderly, often remember the history of the building they are in and view it with suspicion. Frequently they regard hospitalization there as a death sentence ('they used to come here to die, you know'). Similarly staff working in old premises seem to favour tradition. They may follow inflexible, hierarchical working practices, based on out-dated models and systems (see Chapters 4 and 5). One of the reasons for this may be due to the buildings themselves. Often, these house old, established, bureaucratic institutions whilst newer hospitals, for example, house younger organizations. Older systems may be reluctant to recognize those professions whose history is fairly recent (see Chapter 3). Some staff even oppose any attempts at innovation, however well-intentioned.

All these features are relevant for anyone trying vainly to generate an enthusiastic team approach. Sometimes (although not always) it is the environment itself, which proves the stumbling block. It creates a negative, stagnant atmosphere affecting the attitudes and motivation of staff. Again, this is another problem to which there is no easy solution. Nevertheless recognizing the situation for what it is may prevent the disillusioned individual from blaming herself, or others, or both.

Those who work in more modern premises, such as a recently built district general hospital or modern health centre, gain definite advantages. The environment itself assists teamwork even before it is put into practice. Close location between departments, for example, allows informal access and easy contact between individuals. This provides opportunities for discussion and joint treatment sessions if necessary (see the case histories in Chapter 7). Regular contact promotes the growth of working relationships and the exchange of ideas.

A further practical issue arising from previous chapters concerns the notion of leader of the team. Some centres already use a 'key worker' to coordinate the activities of the various members of staff (see Chapter 2; Garner, 1990, pp. 8, 94; and the MNDA newsletter mentioned above). In my experience this enlightened policy is the exception rather than the rule in most hospitals. Usually the consultant heads the troupe because he holds overall responsibility for the patient, but his presence can have a negative influence on both patients and other staff. Hopkins Rintala *et al.* (1986) analysed the speech used during ward rounds in a rehabilitation hospital. They report that physicians spoke more (41%) and made more authoritative statements (62%) than did staff from any other discipline. Patients contributed only 9% of the discussion and made less than 1% of authoritative statements. Furthermore, discussion about physical matters overshadowed psychological needs.

Their findings verify the reports by patients themselves in Chapter 2. Frequently their emotional and social needs are ignored. These facts have implications for those who work with social workers and clinical psychologists. Often these are the individuals best equipped to assume the mantle of key worker. They have the opportunity and training to look at the patient as a whole, often at home in the community after discharge.

It is up to each professional to ensure that the key worker knows what she can offer the patient. This means getting to know the key worker well. This, in turn, may entail conscious efforts to arrange contact and opportunities for discussion and exchange of information. The key worker cannot replace the expertise of another specialist, but she needs to have the opportunity to learn what this expertise is. Otherwise she will be unable to call in the correct professional at the right time.

Another practical suggestion is the use of a team booklet for both patients and staff. This would improve communication on all sides. Staff would know who was involved with the patient. Patients would be better informed about the team directing their care. Such a booklet would need to be updated regularly as staff changed and someone would need to be in charge of this.

Identification of personnel can improve communication. Indeed in some wards, particularly those operating primary nursing (see Chapter 5), individual staff are identified by photograph and name at the entrance to the ward. Perhaps other team members could be included on this too – particularly if they had regular contact with that particular ward. The use of a team booklet like this follows the principles of the 'Patient's

Charter' in the UK. This establishes patients' rights and aims to inform them both of services provided and how to obtain further information.

Training issues

The conclusions drawn from Chapter 6 provide further thought for discussion. An important issue there was the closer liaison and contact between the managers and teaching staff of different disciplines. This could have further advantages – particularly access by members of one profession to the literature of another. In my own experience both tutors and managers of different professions have little knowledge of the textbooks available in other disciplines. This is unfortunate because these often contain useful information. Relevant professional issues and practical expertise (for example the correct handwashing procedure – see Chapter 6) are just two examples. Furthermore, such texts often contain vital information hidden to anyone who is not a member of that profession. Many good nursing textbooks include an exhaustive list of useful names, addresses and contact numbers of a variety of groups, for example the Carers National Association and the self-help groups listed in Chapter 2. Dittmar (1989) and Royle and Wash (1992) are two such works. Their pages probably reflect the more holistic nature of nursing, sometimes overlooked by the specialist professionals. Similarly Baldwin and Hopcroft's 'Handbook for Housemen' (1987) contains useful practical details, for example the meaning of various abbreviations in the medical notes.

Reading the literature from other professions promotes an understanding of their roles. It gives an insight into the problems they experience and the range of their expertise. Accessible, user-friendly texts with a minimum of jargon are particularly helpful. There is a need for individual professions to produce basic works like this to assist the training and education of their colleagues from other disciplines. Lynch and Grigogono (1991) have written an excellent book on strokes and head injuries which can be easily understood by those who are not trained physiotherapists. Similarly works in the 'Therapy in Practice' series, published by Chapman and Hall in London, can be understood by individuals from a wide range of disciplines. More are needed if information between the professions is to be shared and accessed easily. Tutors and lecturers should be aware of this literature and should highlight relevant texts for their students. Sharing information which can be read easily may assist professionals in their work and promote team spirit. Indeed some of the literature from the self-help groups already achieves this (see Chapter 2).

There are further recommendations to be drawn about training and education;. Chapter 6 suggested joint work between students of different disciplines. Discussion centred around sharing of lectures and practical work. This leads to comments about the examination system itself. Most professional bodies award qualifications on the basis of the ability to answer essay-type questions as part of a written examination. There are usually several papers which need to be passed. Occasionally marks are awarded on the basis of course work or project work.

Nevertheless both the exam system and ongoing evaluation militate against teamwork. This is because they do not directly reward individuals for conferring or for trying to solve problems jointly by sharing their expertise. Instead marks are awarded for individual excellence. Students gain prestige and, in many cases, better employment opportunities by obtaining higher grades and credits than their peers. In this way they are encouraged to compete against one another rather than gain rewards by showing their ability to work together. This is unfortunate because negotiation and collaboration with others are vital for teamwork in the future.

This individualistic, competitive approach deserves comparison with the practices of other cultures – particularly the Japanese. Their motor industry, for example, rewards those workers who are able to tackle a problem together, seeing it through to the end. Workers often need to share expertise and learn from one another. Indeed collaboration like this is admired, favoured characteristics including an ability to share knowledge constructively and work within a group. Although the Japanese education system stresses individual competition, in society and the workplace, the group is considered more important. This contrasts sharply with our own testing system which uses individual final examinations and percentage marks. These conspire against teamwork by fostering individual excellence in the face of competition, rather than problem solving through collaboration.

It is hard to envisage a scenario where joint work between, for example, students of nursing and occupational therapy carry greater reward than outstanding individual exam results by either one working on their own. Obviously each discipline still needs to examine its characteristic core skills. Nevertheless some form of joint evaluation does deserve consideration, particularly if professions wish to foster teamwork in their prospective qualified workers.

A further important point about training and education concerns levels of expertise and knowledge. Obviously anyone working in a team needs to know what they are talking about with regard to their own profession. This knowledge is necessary for two reasons. They need to know their own subject if they are to offer valuable specialist expertise to the team as a whole. In addition this knowledge promotes respect in their fellow members. A problem arises when knowledge within a discipline advances and changes and practices alter. Chapter six gives an example of this in physiotherapy where 'the compensatory approach' to hemiplegia gave way to other strategies.

Numerous further examples exist in other professions and controversy arises even in contemporary textbooks. Consider the nursing practice of 'last offices' performed on the body of a patient who has died. Pritchard and David (1988) state that dressings and drainage tubes should be removed. Clarke (1991), however, maintains that any dressings should be left undisturbed, fresh ones being placed over them if any seepage had occurred. If members of one profession have different views about certain practices and techniques, then there is more chance of confusion for fellow team members. Expertise is constantly advancing, therefore current standards and techniques need to be defined. Professionals, therefore, need to know their own standards. This means that professional bodies and managerial staff need to provide specific guidelines. Departmental policies are a step in the right direction.

Issues of personality and emotion

Several books and articles describe the influence of personality on team work. Nieuwenhuis (1990, p. 7), for example, describes a programme of practical joint treatment activities for a young head-injured victim. These are carried out together by a physiotherapist, an occupational therapist and a speech and language therapist. Nieuwenhuis attributes success, amongst other factors, to the three compatible 'non-territorial' personalities of those involved. Similarly, Fussey and Giles (1988, p. 185) state that professional ego must take second place in treatment of the severely brain-injured adult (see also Smyth, 1990; Squires, 1988 and Garner, 1990).

The following sections contain practical suggestions for fostering non-territorial attitudes at work. They are based directly on clinical experience,. No doubt they are not new to many workers. Nevertheless, stating certain obvious steps offers positive reinforcement and encouragement to individuals at work. Firstly, an informal visit to another department early on after starting a job can pay dividends. Other staff may have heard about someone's arrival through the grapevine but may have had no time to establish contact. Indeed they may expect this to come from the newcomer, with support from her in-line manager. Unfortunately, lack of time, lack of support, and ignorance may prevent the initial contact being made. This deficiency may never be recompensed.

The situation is similar to meeting new neighbours after moving into a new home. Introductions are feasible in the UK for 4–5 weeks after the newcomers arrive but thereafter the opportunity declines. The chance of establishing friendly relations is lost. Indeed subsequent contact can often be a source of stress and embarrassment. Similarly, at work, a timely visit early on can foster friendly relations, creating fertile ground for joint contact in the future. Initial introductions may prove more beneficial in the long run than tackling head on a heavy, daunting caseload. For one thing, the regular staff in the other departments are able to put a face to a name. For another, they may be more inclined to continue the contact over the following weeks and provide help and support for joint problems when required.

Another action which assists friendly relations is to show a genuine interest in the practices of fellow professionals. This is equally as important as advertising personal professional expertise. It may entail, for example, enquiring about the organization of the ward in a hospital, the working hours of community colleagues and, later on, the current favoured method of treatment for a particular patient. Sharing knowledge like this can help to avoid those defensive professional barriers behind which individuals may hide. Unfortunately these often heighten the ignorance surrounding what another discipline actually does. This negative response is often based on unfamiliarity and contributes to a 'not invented here' syndrome. This reflects resistance to change, a refusal to recognize the value of anything unless it comes from a known and trusted source. Showing a healthy interest and sharing information may promote the development and acceptance of new ideas thereby increasing joint expertise.

It is often helpful to try to empathize with the pressures experienced by other professionals (see Chapter 3). Frequently the stresses of one's own job take precedence over those of anyone else. Sometimes, however, a sympathetic word to another person actually reduces the tension for both involved. A sense of humour undoubtedly helps; in fact the funny side of the job, shared with others, is often the best remembered part.

Hamdy *et al.* (1990, p. 136) stress the importance of both 'professional stroking' from colleagues and liking the people round about. Staff from any discipline and of any rank and grade have equal roles to play. The unqualified auxiliary nurse, ward receptionist, housekeeper or domestic may be just as vital as the highly trained doctor because of their invaluable sense of humour and willingness to help. Nevertheless lack of self confidence and low status may obscure their perception of their own value. Hence they, too, need encouragement and 'stroking' from those with whom they come into contact. Compliments and thanks contribute to a positive team spirit. They are essential when someone has helped (for example lifting a patient up the bed for therapy) or has carried out instructions which were left (for example positioning the patient in a particular way).

Empathizing with patient and family is equally important. The background literature of the self-help groups surveyed for Chapter 2 suggests that relatives frequently notice clinically irrelevant points. In other words, they tend to focus on something which they assume indicates that the patient's condition has improved, although it may be insignificant to the specialist professional. Her training and experience may tell her that the eventual prognosis remains the same. The dysphasic patient, for example, who produces a whole phrase one day (to the

delight of his family) may never be able to repeat it. Similarly, the hemiplegic patient who shows a slight and brief automatic associated reaction in moving his affected foot may nonetheless never walk again.

The problem for the professional stems from her wealth of knowledge. To her, the clinical insignificance of the patient's performance may be glaringly obvious. However this is only because she is now an expert in her field. Remembering how little you knew in the beginning (the plight of most patients and relatives) must become an important consideration. This provides a base for empathy and an appropriate response.

SUMMARY

My impression is that, in several cases, teamwork can be easier in hospital than in the community. A variety of factors contribute to this. In hospital, individuals of different professions are at least located on the same site. Therefore access to each other may be easier. Furthermore they are already part of an established hierarchical structure within the hospital system. Although departments may not understand each others' roles, they may at least be aware of each others' existence. This provides a basis on which to work.

Community team work, on the other hand, is much more difficult. Jones (1992) outlines the problems facing the community physiotherapist. These are easily applicable to any community professional. They include psychological, social and environmental problems. In addition there may be difficulties in communicating with others, situations where the actual diagnosis is unclear (see Chapter 8 of this book for an example of this) and the loneliness inherent in having to work in isolation. There are various strategies for coping with these problems (see Jones, 1992).

Jones' remarks and my own experience suggest that success in the community is perhaps more difficult to achieve than in hospital. Again, there are several reasons for this. The community professional has less contact with others than her hospital peers. Therefore opportunities for praise and 'professional stroking' are fewer. Similarly any success she achieves will have a limited audience – perhaps only the patient and his family. This means that working in the community often brings less kudos in some situations than working in a specialist, highly renowned, technological unit such as hospital neurology and neurosurgery.

Facts like these partly explain Jones' (1992) recommendation that the community professional should have had at least 3 years experience since qualifying. Without these, she might be unable to cope with all the pressures and the possible, sometimes inevitable, lack of support. Unfortunately it is hospital success stories which receive publicity and reward. Success in the community may be harder to define. Nevertheless the community worker may put in just as much effort; more, in some cases, due to the circumstances under which she has to work.

A helpful development would be greater recognition for community teamwork. This has to come from the professionals involved because no one else will be able to advertise the issue. It entails adopting a higher profile in order to raise interest and awareness. One way of doing this is for professionals to write down their experiences for others to read. This does not require an academic, literary training but merely the ability to construct reports – a skill learnt during most professional training. A wide range of journals and papers are available, for example *Nursing Times* and *Therapy Weekly*. These usually welcome information which may be of interest to readers and any medical library will be able to give an exhaustive list of other potential sources. Hewlett (1990) is an excellent reference book and gives other useful information.

The content of individual reports and articles need be neither erudite, technical nor contain momentous life-saving discoveries. Straightforward, jargon free, user-friendly descriptions of about 1000–2000 words are quite enough. They are always refreshing, especially if they have been written by one professional for people who belong to different disciplines. Furthermore they need not necessarily involve statistically significant, quantitative, objective findings, so admired by the medical profession. They simply need to contain something of interest.

Indeed a rigorous scientific approach is not always appropriate when evaluating patient/relative satisfaction or the success of multidisciplinary activity. In any case, there are ethical questions surrounding the traditional, medical approach to research (see Chapters 2 and 6). Neuberger (1992), in a report on ethics and health care, argues that sick people should not be subjected to unnecessary research. Others have voiced this concern too. 'It is necessary to consider the significance of outcome for the patient, rather than the statistical significance required for publication in learned journals. The central consideration must be quality of life for the patient and his or her family' (Fussey and Giles, 1988, p. 198).

Finally, in some areas advanced technology has promoted teamwork. This is not restricted to health care alone. A television programme ('Before Babel: The First Spoken Language', *Horizon*, BBC2, April 1992) highlighted the way in which genetics, linguistics, archeology and anthropology had worked together to confirm tentative historical knowledge. The discussion centred around the origins of the Basques and the Basque language in Europe. Following detailed language analysis, linguists suggest that Basque is historically independent and isolated from other languages. Geneticists are able to confirm this hypothesis. Their detailed analysis concludes that the Basque people themselves are genetically distinct. Incidentally, analyses also indicated that the first humans came out of Africa.

This is an example, outside health care, of teamwork which relies heavily on advanced technological expertise. Each field needed the help of the other to confirm their investigations. Pooling of experience and skills and technological know-how promoted the progress of knowledge itself. The same process occurs frequently in health care, particularly in specialist areas which are forced to share their technological expertise. One example is the development of new communication aids, blending the skills of computer experts, occupational therapists and speech and language therapists. Others include the investigation of dysphagia, using the expertise of radiologists and speech and language therapists, and computerized ward notes, sharing the knowledge of doctors and nurses. Knowledge in each field progresses because individuals from separate disciplines begin to pool their skills and expertise.

Such examples imply that advanced technology may inspire teamwork by acting as a catalyst. Individuals may liaise more easily when forced to collaborate with the development of technical expertise in different fields. The initial 'threat' posed by new technology may actually provide improved opportunities for cooperation. This may be one of the reasons which make teamwork in hospital easier to achieve, at least initially, than teamwork in the community. Teaching hospitals, in particular, tend to have readier access to technology than do isolated community centres. Therefore their staff have contact and liaison forced upon them.

The situation may change. The use of technology itself may slow down as the cost rises. Hence the rate of teamwork, already known to enhance patient care, may also decelerate. Unfortunately any such dwindling in teamwork may detract from care of the patient as a whole. This reinforces the need to advertise situations where disciplines manage to work well together, despite the acclaimed difficulties. High-tech expertise is not a necessary condition for cooperation, but knowledge about one another definitely is. Increased mutual knowledge will reduce the situations where 'we each secretly believe that our discipline has the most to offer' (Fussey and Giles, 1988, p. 184) and '. . . each discipline thinks it understands exactly what all the other disciplines do' (Thomas, 1988, p. 123).

This book has tried to share knowledge between the professions and thereby promote understanding between those who work with the adult with acquired neurological brain damage. Hopefully it has given some insight into what different individuals do. This may help to foster the ultimate aim of all team members – namely to improve the quality of care for the patient, the customer of the services offered by the team.

Appendix A: Useful addresses

Every effort has been made to ensure that the following addresses and telephone numbers are current and correct.

ADDRESSES IN THE UK

Alzheimer's Disease Society
158–160 Balham High Road
London SW12 9BN
Tel: 081 675 6557

British Dietetic Association
7th Floor
Elizabeth House
Suffolk Street
Queensway
Birmingham B1 1LS
Tel: 021 6161091

British Medical Association (BMA)
BMA House
Tavistock Square
London WC1H 9JP
Tel: 071 383 6101

Carers National Association
29 Chilworth Mews
London
W2 3RG
Tel: 071 724 7776

Clinical Psychological Division
The British Psychological Society
St. Andrews House
48 Princess Road East
Leicester LE1 7DR
Tel: 0533 549568

College of Occupational Therapists
6–8 Marshalsea Road
Southwark
London SE1 1HL
Tel: 071 357 6480

Friedreich's Ataxia Group
Burleigh Lodge
Knowle Lane
Cranleigh
Surrey GU6 8RD

Guillain–Barré Syndrome Support Group
Foxley
Holdingham
Sleaford
Lincs NG34 8NR
Tel: 0529 304615

Headway
7 King Edward Street
Nottingham NG1 1EW
Tel: 0602 240 800

Huntingdon's Disease Association
108 Battersea High Street
London SW11 3HP
Tel: 071 223 7000

Motor Neurone Disease Association
PO Box 246
Northampton NN1 2PR
Tel: 0604 250505

Multiple Sclerosis Society of Great Britain and Northern Ireland
25 Effie Road
Fulham
London SW6 1EE
Tel: 071 736 6267

Myaesthenia Gravis Association
Keynes House
77 Nottingham Road
Derby DE1 3QS
Tel: 0332 290219

Parkinson's Disease Society
22 Upper Woburn Place
London WC1H 0RA
Tel: 071 383 3513

Royal College of Nursing of the United Kingdom (RCN)
20 Cavendish Square
London W1M 0AB
Tel: 071 409 3333

Royal College of Nursing and Council of Nurses of the United Kingdom (RCN) Scotland
44 Heriot Row
Edinburgh EH3 6EY

Royal College of Nursing and National Council of Nurses of the United Kingdom (RCN) Welsh Board
Ty Maeth
King George V Drive
East Cardiff CF4 4XZ

Stroke Association
CHSA House
123/127 Whitecross Street
London EC1Y 8JJ
Tel: 071 490 7999

The Central Council for Education and Training in Social Work Information Service
Derbyshire House
St Chad's Street
London WC1H 8AD

The Chartered Society of Physiotherapy
14 Bedford Row
London WC1R 4ED
Tel: 071 242 1941

The College of Speech and Language Therapists
7 Bath Place
Rivington Street
London EC2A 3DR
Tel: 071 613 3855

ADDRESSES IN THE USA

American Nurses' Association, Inc.
Suite 500
2420 Pershing Road
Kansas City, Missouri 64108
Tel: 1913 474 5720

Amyotrophic Lateral Sclerosis Association
15300 Ventura Blvd., Suite 315
Sherman Oaks, CA 91403
Tel: 818 990 2151

Myaesthenia Gravis Foundation, Inc.
53 W. Jackson Blvd., Suite 909
Chicago, IL 60604
Tel: 312 427 6252

National Head Injury Foundation
333 Turnpike Road
Southborough, MA 01772
Tel: 617 485 9950

National Multiple Sclerosis Society
205 East 42 Street
New York, NY 10017–5706
Tel: 212 986 3240

Parkinson's Disease Foundation
William Black Medical Research Building Columbia-Presbyterian Medical Center
650 West 168th Street
New York, NY 10032
Tel: 212 923 4700

Stroke Clubs International
805–12th Street
Galveston, TX 775500

The American Parkinson Disease Association
60 Bay Street
Staten Island, NY 10301
Tel: 212 732 9550

Appendix B: Glossary

ACTH (adrenocorticotrophic hormone) A hormone synthesized and stored in the anterior pituitary gland, controlling the secretion of corticosteroid hormones from the adrenal gland.

Alzheimer's disease A progressive form of dementia occurring in middle age or later, for which there is no cure. It is associated with diffuse degeneration of the brain.

Angioma A knot of distended blood vessels overlying and compressing the surface of the brain.

Anoxia A condition in which the tissues of the body receive inadequate amounts of oxygen.

Arachnoid mater The middle of the three membranes covering the brain and spinal cord.

Ataxia The shaky movements and unsteady gait that result from the brain's failure to regulate the body's posture and the strength and direction of limb movements.

Autonomic system The part of the nervous system responsible for the control of bodily functions which are not consciously directed. This includes regular beating of the heart, intestinal movements, sweating, salivation etc.

Barrier nursing The nursing care of an infectious patient in isolation from other patients to prevent the spread of infection.

Basal ganglia Several large masses of grey matter embedded deep within the white matter of the cerebrum. They include the *caudate* and the *lenticular nuclei* (together known as the *corpus striatum*) and the *amygdaloid nucleus*. The lenticular nucleus consists of the *putamen* and the *globus pallidus*. The basal ganglia are involved with the regulation of voluntary movements at a subconscious level.

Behaviourism A theory of learning in which observable behaviour is explained in terms of the individual's interaction with the environment. His responses are a product of the stimuli to which he is exposed.

Behaviour modification The use of structured programmes, including reinforcements, to modify behaviour. This works either by removing unwanted behaviour or by promoting positive behaviour.

Biomedical approach An approach to health care which views individuals as made up of physical, measurable systems. Disease occurs when a system malfunctions. Subsequent treatment aims to improve and cure, if possible, the malfunction in that system. This approach favours objective, scientific data.

Bobath concept A bilateral approach to the treatment of hemiplegia or spasticity, involving inhibition of unwanted muscle patterns and facilitation of automatic reactions (righting, equilibrium and protective extension).

Bradykinesia Slowness of movement.

Brainstem The enlarged extension upwards within the skull of the spinal cord. It consists of the medulla oblongata, the pons and the midbrain.

Cerebellum The largest part of the hindbrain, bulging back behind the pons and the medulla oblongata and overhung by the occipital lobes of the cerebrum.

Cerebral aneurysm A balloon-like swelling in the wall of an artery in the brain, due to disease or congenital deficiency.

Cerebral oedema The excessive accumulation of fluid in the brain.

Chorea Jerky involuntary movement, particularly affecting the shoulders, hips and face. Symptoms are due to disease of the basal ganglia.

Conductive education A highly structured and formal treatment method used with cerebral palsied children and adults with neurological impairment. Pioneered in Hungary, it concentrates on functional tasks, with intensive treatment programmes tailored to suit each individual.

Counselling The use of client-centred techniques which help individuals to identify problems, feelings or conflicts and reach a solution or decision about them.

CT scan (CAT scan) A specialist X-ray showing an integrated three-dimensional image of the soft structures of the body, particularly the brain.

Dementia A chronic or persistent disorder of the mental processes due to organic brain disease. It is marked by memory disorders, changes in personality, deterioration in personal care, impaired reasoning ability and disorientation.

Diplopia Double vision.

Dysarthria A speech disorder resulting from disturbance of neuromuscular control. It is caused by damage to the central nervous system or peripheral nervous system. It also occurs in association with some muscle diseases. Weakness, incoordination or altered muscle tone create speech which may have faulty articulation, respiration, voicing, resonance or intonation.

Dysphagia Difficulty in swallowing.

Dysphasia A disorder of processing and formulating language. Patients have difficulty understanding what is said and what they read. They also have difficulty in recalling the vocabulary and grammatical structures necessary for producing speech and in writing.

Dura (Dura Mater) The thickest and outermost of the three meninges (membranes) surrounding the brain and spinal cord.

Encephalitis Inflammation of the brain.

Extradural haematoma A haematoma (or blood clot) caused by tearing of the middle meningeal artery as a result of injury to the head.

Extrapyramidal system The system of nerve tracts and pathways connecting the cerebral cortex, basal ganglia, thalamus, cerebellum, reticular formation and spinal neurones in complex circuits not included in the pyramidal system. The extrapyramidal system is concerned with the regulation of stereotyped reflex muscular movements.

Friedreich's Ataxia An inherited disorder appearing first in adolescence. It has features of cerebellar ataxia, together with spasticity of the limbs.

Glasgow Coma Scale A scale which categorizes the levels of responsiveness after head injury.

Global dysphasia Severe impairment in all areas of speech and language function (i.e. understanding, speaking, reading and writing).

Guillain–Barré syndrome An acute distress of the nervous system involving the spinal nerve roots, peripheral nerve and cranial nerves.

Haemorrhage The escape of blood from a ruptured blood vessel.

Hemianopia Loss of vision for one half of the visual field of one or both eyes.

Hemiplegia Paralysis of one side of the body.

Homonymous hemianopia Blindness in the corresponding (right or left) field of vision of each eye.

Humanist approach An approach to health care which stresses the individual as a whole and the way in which body and mind interact.

Huntingdon's Chorea An inherited form of chorea (jerky involuntary movement) in which the involuntary movements are accompanied by progressive dementia. There is widespread neuronal degeneration throughout the brain.

Hydrocephalus An abnormal increase in the amount of cerebrospinal fluid within the ventricles of the brain.

Hyperbaric oxygen treatment Treatment for multiple sclerosis which increases the oxygen in the body by placing the patient in an atmosphere of increased pressure.

Hyper-reflexic Showing exaggerated reflex responses.

Hypertonic Showing an abnormal increase in tonicity.

Hypokinesia Poverty of movement.

Hypoxia A deficiency of oxygen in the tissues.

Incidence/prevalence of a disease Incidence refers to the number of new cases diagnosed within a particular period, usually a year. Prevalence refers to the number of cases occurring in a population at a particular point in time, usually measured on a particular day, such as the 1st of January.

Intention tremor Tremor that occurs when a patient with disease of the cerebellum tries to touch an object.

Intubation Passage of an oro- or nasotracheal tube for anaesthesia or for control of pulmonary ventilation.

Ischaemia An inadequate flow of blood to a part of the body.

Johnstone Concept of Rehabilitation A method for the treatment of stroke developed by Margaret Johnstone in the 1970s.

Kernig's sign A symptom of meningitis in which the patient is unable to extend his legs at the knee when the thighs are held at a right angle to the body.

Lumbar puncture A procedure in which cerebrospinal fluid is drawn for diagnostic purposes by means of a hollow needle inserted into the subarachnoid region of the lower back (usually between the third and fourth lumbar vertebrae).

Meninges The three connective membranes that line the skull and vertebral canal and enclose the brain and spinal cord. They are known, respectively, as the dura mater, the arachnoid mater and the pia mater.

Meningitis An inflammation of the meninges due to viral or bacterial infection.

Motor learning programme A physiotherapy treatment which teaches the patient specific functional tasks by breaking these down into their constituent parts.

Motor neurone disease A progressive degenerative disease of the motor system occurring in middle age and causing muscle wasting and weakness. It primarily affects the cells of the anterior horn of the spinal cord, the motor nuclei in the brainstem and the corticospinal fibres.

MPTP 1-methyl–4–phenyl–1,2,3,6-tetrahydropyridine: a chemical that aggravates/causes Parkinsonism.

Multiple sclerosis A chronic disease of the nervous system affecting young and middle-aged adults. The myelin sheaths surrounding nerves in the brain and spinal cord are damaged, which affects the function of the nerves involved.

Myaesthenia gravis A chronic disease marked by abnormal fatigability and weakness of selected muscles.

Neurodevelopmental approach An approach to health care which assumes that growth and change occur in recognized stages, related to the acquisition of sensori-motor skills.

Neuromuscular junction The meeting point of a motor nerve fibre and the muscle fibre that it supplies. It consists of a minute gap across which a neurotransmitter must diffuse from the nerve to trigger contraction of the muscle.

Neurostransmitter A chemical substance, such as acetycholine, released from nerve endings to transmit impulses across syapses (gaps between neurones) to other nerves – and across the minute gaps between the nerves and the muscles or glands that they supply.

Nursing process An individualized problem-solving approach to the nursing care of patients. It involves four stages: assessment (of the patient's problems), planning (how to resolve them), implementation (of the plans) and evaluation (of their success).

Nystagmus Rapid involuntary movements of the eyes that may be from side to side, up and down, or rotatory.

Papilloedema Swelling of the optic disc.

Paresis Muscular weakness caused by disease of or damage to the nervous system.

Parkinsonism A disorder of middle-aged and elderly people characterized by tremor, rigidity and a poverty of spontaneous movements. Other features include an expressionless face and a monotonous voice. The disease affects the basal ganglia of the brain.

Perceptual training Techniques designed to train or re-educate perceptual functions such as discriminations of size, form, colour, laterality etc.

Percutaneous endoscopic gastrostomy (P.E.G.) The insertion through the skin of a small tube directly into the stomach to allow food and fluid to be poured in. This tube may remain permanently in situ, all meals being given through it. It can also be removed once the patient is able to fulfill his nutritional requirements by eating and drinking normally.

Persistent vegetative state A state during the recovery from deep coma, usually after a head injury. The patient is awake, may follow people with his eyes and respond in a limited way to primitive postural and reflex movements without any awareness of the environment or real need.

Pes cavus An excessively arched foot, giving an unnaturally high instep.

Photophobia An abnormal intolerance of light. Exposure to it produces intense discomfort of the eyes with tight contraction of the eyelids.

POMR (Problem orientated medical recording) A way of recording information about patients' problems and ensuing intervention in a logical format.

Primary health care team A group of professionals who work together to provide health care outside a hospital setting.

Proprioceptive neuromuscular facilitation A treatment technique for neurological damage which uses positioning and patterns of movement in developmental sequence. It emphasizes sensory input as a way of maximizing motor output.

Ptosis Drooping of the upper eyelid.

Raised intracranial pressure A rise in pressure caused by an increase in the volume of the intracranial contents.

Reality orientation A treatment method used with dementing or brain damaged individuals. It cues them into awareness of current time, place, persons and circumstances.

Reticular formation A network of nerve pathways and nuclei throughout the brainstem, connecting motor and sensory nerves to and from the spinal cord, the cerebellum and the cerebrum, and the cranial nerves.

Rigidity Resistance to the passive movement of a limb that persists throughout its range.

Rood approach A treatment method for stroke developed by an American called Margaret Rood. It involves sensory stimulation, particularly tactile stimulation.

Spasticity Resistance to the passive movement of a limb that is maximal at the beginning of the movement and gives way as more pressure is applied.

Stroke Serious, spontaneous disturbance of the blood supply to the brain, caused by ischaemia or haemorrhage.

Subdural haematoma A haematoma (or blood clot) caused by tearing of the veins where they cross the space beneath the dura in the brain.

Tone The normal state of partial contraction of a resting muscle.

Tonicity The normal state of slight contraction, or readiness to contract, of healthy muscle fibres.

Ventilator Equipment that is manually or mechanically operated to maintain a flow or air into and out of the lungs of a patient who is unable to breathe normally.

Bibliography

Aggleton, P. and Chalmers, H. (1986) *Nursing Models and the Nursing Process*, London, Macmillan Education.

Allen, C. M. C., Harrison, M. J. G. and Wade, D. T. (1988) *The Management of Acute Stroke*, Kent, Castle House Publications.

Anon (Summer 1990) The Day Life Changed. *Headway News* p. 4., Nottingham, Headway, National Head Injuries Association.

Ashworth, B. and Saunders, M. (1985) *Management of Neurological Disorders*, 2nd edn, London, Butterworths.

Atkinson, R. L., Atkinson, R. C., Smith, E. E., Bem, D. J. and Hilgard, E. R. (1990) *Introduction to Psychology*, 10th edn, New York, Harcourt Brace.

Baker, M. and McCall, B. (1991) The Parkinson's Disease Society. In Caird, F. I. (ed.) *Rehabilitation in Parkinson's Disease*, pp. 120–7, London, Chapman and Hall.

Baldwin, D. and Hopcroft, K. (1987) *A Handbook for Housemen*, Oxford, Blackwell Scientific Publications.

Banks, S. (1990) Consider the Mind as Well as the Body. *Professional Nurse*, October, pp. 9–14.

Barber, J. and Kratz, C. (1980) (eds) *Towards Team Care*, London, Churchill Livingstone.

Beck, A. T. (1988) *Beck Depression Inventory*, Sidcup, Kent, The Psychological Corporation Limited.

Bickerstaff, E. R. (1978) *Neurology*, 3rd edn, London, Hodder and Stoughton.

Bishop, J., Caygill, D., Mace, C. *et al.* (1990) Disabled for a Day. *Nursing Times*, **86** (21), 66–67.

Brandstater, M. E. and Basmajian, J. V. (1987) (eds) *Stroke Rehabilitation*, Baltimore, USA, Williams and Wilkins.

Brooks, D. N. (1984) *Closed Head Injury: Psychological, Social and Family Consequences*, Oxford, Oxford University Press.

Brooks, D. N., Campsie, L., Symington, C., Beattie, A. and Mckinlay, W. (1986) The Five Year Outcome of Severe Blunt Head Injury: A Relative's View. *Journal of Neurology, Neurosurgery and Psychiatry*, **49**, 764–70.

Bukowski, L., Bonavolonta, M., Keehn, M. T. and Morgan, K. A. (1986) Interdisciplinary Roles in Stroke Care. *Nursing Clinics of North America*, **21** (2), 359–74.

Burnard, P. (1989) *Counselling Skills for Health Professionals*, London, Chapman and Hall.

Burnard, P. (1990) 'Learning from Experience: Nurse Tutors' and Student Nurses' Perceptions of Experimental Learning' Ph.D. Thesis, Cardiff, School of Nursing Studies, University of Wales College of Medicine.

Cadwaller, H. (1989) Setting the Seal of Standards. *Nursing Times*, **85** (37), 70–71.

Caird, F. I. (1991) (ed.) *Rehabilitation in Parkinson's Disease*, London, Chapman and Hall.

Cantrell, T. (1988) The Young Adult with Neurological Disabilities. In Goodwill, C. J. and Chamberlain, M. A. (eds) *Rehabilitation of the Physically Disabled Adult*, pp. 287–307, London, Croom Helm.

Cantrell, E. G. and Dawson, J. (1983) Young Disabled in the Community. In Barbenel, J., Forbes, C. D. and Lowe, G. D. O. (eds) *Pressure Sores*, London, Macmillan.

Capra, F. (1982) *The Turning Point*, London, Fontana.

Carpenter, M. (1980) Asylum Nursing Before 1914: A Chapter in the History of Labour. In Davis, C. (ed.) *Rewriting Nursing History*, pp. 123–46, London, Croom Helm.

Carr, J. H. and Shepherd, R. B. (1980) *Physiotherapy in Disorders of the Brain*, London, William Heinemann Medical Books.

Chesson, R. (1992) Research on a Shoestring. *Therapy Weekly* **19** (19), 7.

Carr-Saunders, A. M. and Wilson, P. A. (1933) *The Professions*, London, Cass.

Clarke, M. (1991) *Practical Nursing*, 14th edn, London, Baillière Tindall.

Cochrane, G. M. (1987) (ed.) *The Management of Motor Neurone Disease*, Edinburgh, Churchill Livingstone.

Cole, J. (1986) A Word in your Ear. *Nursing Times*, September 10, **53** pp.

Collen, F. M., Wade, D. T., Robb, G. F. and Bradshaw, C. M. (1991) The Rivermead Mobility Index: A Further Development of the Rivermead Motor Assessment. *Int. Disab. Studies*, **13**, 50–54.

Cumberledge, J. (1986) *Neighbourhood Nursing – A Focus for Care*, London, HMSO.

Deumeurisse, G., Demol, O. and Robaye, E. (1980) Motor Evaluation in Vascular Hemiplegia. *European Neurology* **19**, 382–89.

Dittmar, S. (1989) (ed.) *Rehabilitation Nursing: Process and Application*, St Louis, Missouri, The C. V. Mosby Company.

Eames, P and Wood, R (1989) The Structure and Content of a Head Injury Rehabilitation Service. In Wood, R. and Eames, P. (eds) *Models of Brain Injury Rehabilitation*, pp. 31–47, London, Chapman and Hall.

Edwards, S. and Hanley, J. (1989) Interdisciplinary Activity between Occupational Therapists and Speech Language Pathologists. *Journal of Allied Health*, **18**, (4), 375–87.

Eggers, O. (1988) *Occupational Therapy in the Rehabilitation of Adult Hemiplegia*, London, Heinemann.

Enderby, P. (1988) *Frenchay Dysarthria Assessment*, Windsor, NFER-NELSON.

Enderby, P. M., Wood, V. A., Wade, D. T. and Langton Hewer, R. (1986) The Frenchay Aphasia Screening Test: A short Simple Test for Aphasia Appropriate for Non-Specialists. *International Rehabilitation Medicine* **8**, 166–170.

Enderby, P., Wood, V. and Wade, D. (1987) *Frenchay Aphasia Screening Test*, Windsor, NFER-NELSON.

Freeman, E. A. (1987) (ed.) *The Catastrophe of Coma*, Australia/ New Zealand, David Bateman.

Fussey, I. and Giles, G. M. (1988) (eds) *Rehabilitation of the Severely Brain-Injured Adult: A Practical Approach*, London, Croom Helm.

Garner, R. (1990) *Acute Head Injury*, London, Chapman and Hall.

Goodglass, H. and Kaplan, E. (1972) *The Assessment of Aphasia and Related Disorders*, Philadelphia, Lea and Febiger.

Goodwill, C. J. and Chamberlain, M. A. (1988) (eds) *Rehabili tation of the Physically Disabled Adult*, London, Chapman and Hall.

Granger, C. V. and Gresham, G. E. (1984) (eds) *Functional Assessment in Rehabilitation Medicine*, Baltimore, London, Williams and Wilkins.

Hagedorn, R. (1992) *Occupational Therapy: Foundations for Practice*, London, Churchill Livingstone.

Halligan, P. W., Marshall, J. C. and Wade, D. T. (1989) Visuospatial Neglect: Underlying Factors and Test Sensitivity. *Lancet*, **2**, 908–10.

Hamdy, R. C., Turnbull, J. M., Norman, L. D. and Lancaster, M. M. (1990) *Alzheimer's Disease: A Handbook for Caregivers*, St Louis, Missouri, The C. V. Mosby Company.

Henderson E. J., Morrison, J. A., Young, E. A. and Pentland, B. (1990) The Nurse in Rehabilitation After Severe Brain Injury. *Clinical Rehabilitation* **4**, 167–72.

Hewlett, J. (1990) (ed.) *Keyguide to Information Sources in Paramedical Sciences*, London and New York, Mansell.

Hodkinson, H. M. (1972) Evaluation of a Mental Test Score for Assessment of Mental Impairment in the Elderly. *Age Ageing*, **1**, 233–238.

Hopkins, H. L. (1988) An Historical Perspective on Occupational Therapy. In Hopkins, H. L. and Smith, H. D. (eds.) *Willard and Spackman's Occupational Therapy*, 7th edn, pp. 16–37. Pennsylvania, J. B. Lippincott Company.

Hopkins, H. L. and Smith, H. D. (1983) (eds) *Willard and Spackman's Occupational Therapy*, 6th edn, Pennsylvania, J. B. Lippincott Company.

Hopkins, H. L. and Smith, H. D. (1988) (eds) *Willard and Spackman's Occupational Therapy*, 7th edn, Pennsylvania, J. B. Lippincott Company.

Hopkins Rintala, D., Hanover, D., Alexander, J. L. *et al.* (1986) Team Care: An Analysis of Verbal Behaviour During Patient Rounds in a Rehabilitation Hospital. *Archives of Physical Medicine Rehabilitation*, **67**, 118–22.

Horizon (1992) Before Babel: The First Spoken Language, BBC2, 2 April.

Howard, D., Patterson, K., Franklin, S., Orchard-Lisle, V. and Morton, J. (1985) Treatment of Word Retrieval Deficits in Aphasia. A Comparison of Two Therapy Methods, *Brain* **108**, 817–29.

Howard, D. and Hatfield, F. M. (1987) *Aphasia Therapy: Historical and Contemporary Issues*, Hove, East Sussex, Lawrence Erlbaum Associates.

Hyland, C. and Hyland, K. (1990) Dietetics. In Hewlett, J. (ed.) *Keyguide to Information Sources in Paramedical Sciences*, pp. 88–96, London and New York, Mansell.

Editorial (1992) Doctors Just Don't Have the Right Training. *The Independent*, 14 April.

Isaacs, B. (1982) The Continuing Needs of Stroke Patients. In Rose, F. C. (ed.) *Advances in Stroke Therapy*, pp. 305–312, New York, Raven Press.

Jarman, B. (1988) (ed.) *Primary Care*, London, Heinemann Professional Publishing.

Jennet, B., Teasdale, G., Braakman, R. *et al.* (1979) Prognosis of Patients with Severe Head Injury. *Neurosurgery*, **4** (4), 283–89.

Johnstone, M. (1987) *The Stroke Patient: a Team Approach*, 3rd edn, Edinburgh, Churchill Livingstone.

Jones, F. W. (1992) Stroke Care in the Home. In Downie, P. A. (ed.) *Cash's Textbook of Neurology for Physiotherapists: With a Foreword By Dame Cicely Saunders*, 4th edn, pp. 296–313, London, Wolfe Publishing.

Kaplan, P. E. and Cerullo, L. J. (1986) *Stroke Rehabilitation*, USA, Butterworths.

Kendrick, D (1985) *Kendrick Cognitive Tests for the Elderly*, Windsor, NFER-NELSON.

Kertesz, A. (1982) *Western Aphasia Battery*, Sidcup, Kent, The Psychological Corporation Limited.

King, M., Wieck, L. and Dyer, M. (1981) *Illustrated Manual of Nursing Techniques*, 2nd edn, Philadelphia, J. B. Lippincott.

Lees, M. (1988) The Social and Emotional Consequences of Severe Head Injury: The Social Work Perspective. In Fussey, I. and Giles, G. M. (eds) *Rehabilitation of the Severely Brain-Injured Adult: A Practical Approach*, pp. 166–82, London, Croom Helm.

Levitt, R. and Wall, A. (1992) *The Reorganised National Health Service*, 4th edn, London, Croom Helm.

Lezak, M. D. (1978) Living with the Characterologically Altered Brain-Injured Patient. *Journal of Clinical Psychiatry*, **39**, 592–98.

Livingston, M. G. (1976a) Assessment of Need for Coordinated Approach in Families with Victims of Head Injury. *British Medical Journal*, **293**, 742–44.

Livingston, M. G. (1986b) Head Injury: The Relative's Response. *Brain Injury*, **1**, 8–14.

Logigan, M. K. (1982) (ed.) *Adult Rehabilitation: A Team Approach for Therapists*, Boston, Little, Brown and Co.

Logigan, M. K., Samuels, M. A., Falconer, T. and Zagar, R. (1983) Clinical Exercise Trials for Stroke Patients. *Archives of Physical Medicine and Rehabilitation*, **64**, 364–67.

Lorenz, R. A. and Pichert, J. W. (1986) Impact of Interprofessional Training on Medical Students' Willingness to Accept Clinical Responsibility. *Medical Education*, **20**, 195–200.

Lord, J. P. and Hall, K. H. (1986) Neuromuscular Reeducation Versus Traditional Programs for Stroke Rehabilitation. *Archives of Physical Medicine and Rehabilitation*, **67**, 88–91.

Lynch, M. and Grisogono, V. (1991) *Strokes and Head Injuries: A Guide for Patients, Families, Friends and Carers*, London, John Murray Publishers.

McFarlane, A. (1990) Why Do We Forget Handwashing? *Professional Nurse*, 5 (5), 235–8.

Madsen, M. K., Gresch, A. M., Petterson, B. J. and Taugher M. P. (1988) An Interdisciplinary Clinic for Neurogenically Impaired Adults: A Pilot Project for Educating Students. *Journal of Allied Health*, May, 135–41.

Mahoney, F. I. and Barthel, D. W. (1965) Functional Evaluation: The Barthel Index. *Maryland State Medical J*. **292**, 61–65.

Maloney, F. P., Burks, J. S. and Ringel, S. P. (1985) (eds) *Interdisciplinary Rehabilitation of Multiple Sclerosis and Neuromuscular Disorders*, Philadelphia, J. B. Lippincott Company.

Malzer, R. L. (1988) Patient Performance Level During Inpatient Physical Rehabilitation: Therapist, Nurse, and Patient Perspectives. *Archives of Physical Medicine Rehabilitation*, **69**, May, 363–65.

Mellis, M. (1990) Occupational Therapy. In Hewlett, J. (ed.) *Keyguide to Information Sources In Paramedical Sciences*, pp. 49–72, London and New York, Mansell.

Mody, M. and Nagai, J. (1990) A Multidisciplinary Approach to the Development of Competency Standards and Appropriate Allocation for Patients with Dysphagia. *The American Journal of Occupational Therapy*, **44** (4), 369–72.

Monnot, M. (1988) *From Rage to Courage*, Northfield, Minnestoa, St Denis Press.

Morton, P. (1990a) A Parkinsonian's Special Way of Coping.

In Levin, S. (Ed.) *Coping with Parkinson's Disease*, 2nd edn, pp. 13–14, St Louis, Missouri, American Parkinson Disease Association.

Morton, P. (1990b) The Need to Be Needed. *Hope*, pp. 5–6, London, The Chest, Heart and Stroke Association.

MNDA (Spring 1990) *MNDA Newsletter*, Northampton, Motor Neurone Disease Association.

MNDA (undated) *Motor Neurone Disease: The Role of the Physiotherapist*, Northampton, Motor Neurone Disease Association.

Mulley, G. P. (1985) *Practical Management of Stroke*, London, Croom Helm.

Multiple Sclerosis Society (1990) *Multiple Sclerosis: An Information Pack for Professional Carers*, London, The Multiple Sclerosis Society of Great Britain and Northern Ireland.

Munro, P. (1990) Speech Therapy. In Hewlett, J. (ed.) *Keyguide to Information Sources in Paramedical Sciences*, pp. 97–101, London and New York, Mansell.

Neuberger, J. (1992) *Ethics and Health Care: The Role of Research Ethical Committees in the United Kingdom*, London, King's Fund Institute.

National Council for Vocational Qualifications (1989) *National Council for Vocational Qualifications: Criteria and Procedures*, London, NCVQ.

Nieuwenhuis, R. (1988–1989) Teamwork Within the Community Services. City College, Norwich, NEBSS Diploma

Nieuwenhuis, R. (1989) Breaking the Speech Barrier. *Nursing Times*, **85** (15), 34–36.

Nieuwenhuis, R. (1990) A Team Approach to Head Injury. *Therapy Weekly*, 18 January, p. 7.

Norton, D., Mclaren, R. and Exton-Smith, A. N. (1962) *An Investigation of Geriatric Nursing Problems in Hospital*, London, National Corporation for the Care of Old People.

Orem, D. E. (1980) *Nursing: Concepts of Practice*, 2nd edn, New York, McGraw Hill.

Owen, G. (1977) *Health Visiting*, London, Baillière Tindall.

Oxtoby, M. (1990) Neuro-care Needs More Therapists. *Therapy Weekly*, August 23, p. 11.

Parry, A. (1980) *Physiotherapy Assessment*, 2nd edn, London, Croom Helm.

Pearson, A. and Vaughan, B. (1986) *Nursing Models for Practice*, Oxford, Heinemann Nursing.

190

Pegg, S. (1989–1990) The Storytellers. In *Motor Neurone Disease Association 1989–90*, p. 10, Northampton, Motor Neurone Disease Association.

Phillips, C. (1989) Hand Hygiene. *Nursing Times*, **85** (37), 76–79.

P. J., Mrs (1990) *Headway Newsletter*, 14 March, London, Headway, National Head Injuries Association.

Pritchard, A. and David, J. (1988) (eds) *The Royal Marsden Hospital: Manual of Clinical Nursing Procedures*, 2nd edn, London, Harper and Row.

Ransome, H. (1990) Evaluation and Quality Assurance. In Smyth, L. (ed.) *Practical Physiotherapy with Older People*, pp. 109–53.

Richards, P. (1989) *Learning Medicine 1990: An Informal Guide to a Career in Medicine*, 6th edn, London, British Medical Journal.

Riehl, J. P. and Roy, C. (1980) *Conceptual Models for Nursing Practice*, 2nd edn, New York, Appleton-Century-Crofts.

Robertson, S. J. (1982) *Dysarthria Profile*, Miss Sandra Robertson, 12 Kingsmead, 623 Longbridge Road, Barking, Essex IG11 9BZ.

Robinson, I. (1990) Building the National Register. *MNDA Newsletter*, Summer, p. 2.

Rogers, S (1990) *Things I Wish Someone Had Told Me*, New York, National Multiple Sclerosis Society.

Roper, N., Logan, W. W. and Tierney, A. J. (1980) *The Elements of Nursing*, Edinburgh, Churchill Livingstone.

Routledge, J. and Willson, M. (1992) Joint Does not Mean Generic. *Therapy Weekly*, *19*, (19), 6.

Royle, J. and Walsh, M. (1992) (eds) *Watson's Medical-Surgical Nursing and Related Physiology*, 4th edn, London, Baillière Tindall.

Scott, K. J. (1990) Bereavement Without a Burial. *Alzheimer's Disease Society Newsletter*, November, p. 3.

Senner-Hurley, F. and Lefkowitz, N. G. (1982) Stroke: Speech Language Rehabilitation. In Logigan, M. K. (ed.) *Adult Rehabilitation: a Team Approach for Therapists*, pp. 275–296, Boston, Little, Brown and Company.

Sheikh, K., Smith, D., Meade, T., Brennan, P. and Ide, L. (1980) Assessment of Motor Function in Studies of Chronic Disability, *Rheumatology Rehabilitation.*, **19**, 83–90.

Smyth, L. (1990) *Practical Physiotherapy with Older People*, London, Chapman and Hall.

Somners, T. and Zarit, S. (1985) Seriously Near the Breaking Point. *Generations*.

Spencer, E. A. (1983) Functional Restorastion-Specific Diagnosis. In Hopkins, H. L. and Smith, H. D. (eds) *Willard and Spackman's Occupational Therapy*, 6th edn, pp. 381–446, Philadelphia, J. B. Lippincott.

Squires, A. (1988) (ed.) *Rehabilitation of the Older Patient*, London, Croom Helm.

Squires, A. and Taylor, M. (1988) Assessment of the Older Patient. In Squires, A. (ed.) *Rehabilitation of the Older Patient*, pp. 64–78, London, Croom Helm.

Stevens, R. S. (1989) Stroke Units, *Clinical Rehabilitation*, **3**, 235–37.

Stern, P. H., McDowell, F., Miller, J. M. and Robinson, M. (1970) Effects of Facilitation Exercises in Stroke Rehabilitation. *Archives of Physical Medicine and Rehabilitation*, **51**, 526–31.

Sutcliffe, D. (1990) *Working Alongside Carers*, 9 Milton Crescent, Eastbourne, East Sussex, EB21 1SP, David Sutcliffe.

Talbott, R. (1989) The Brain-Injured Person and the Family., In Wood, R. and Eames. P. (eds) *Models of Brain Injury Rehabilitation*, pp. 3–16, London, Chapman and Hall.

Thomas, L. (1988) The Role of the Nurse in Rehabilitation. In Squires, A. (ed.) *Rehabilitation of the Older Patient*, pp. 123–38, London, Croom Helm.

Thompson, S. B. and Morgan, M. (1990) *Occupational Therapy for Stroke Rehabilitation*, London, Chapman and Hall.

Thurgood, G. (1992) Let's Work Together, Let's Learn Together. *Journal of Advances in Health and Nursing Care*, **1**, (5), 13–40.

Tyerman, R., Tyerman, A., Howard, P. and Hadfield, C. (1986) *The Chessington O.T. Neurological Assessment Battery (COTNAB)*, Nottingham, Nottingham Rehab.

Umphred, D. A. (1985) (ed.) *Neurological Rehabilitation*, vol. 3., St Louis, C. V. Mosby.

University of Leeds (March 1992) Stroke Rehabilitation. *Effective Health Care*, **2**, 1–12.

Voss, D. E. (1967) PNF. *American Journal of Physical Medicine*, **46** (1), 838–98.

Voss, D. E. (1972) Proprioceptive Neuromuscular Facilitation: the PNF Method. In Pearson and Williams (eds) *Physical Therapy Services in Developmental Disabilities*, Springfield, Illinois, Charles C. Thomas.

Wade, D. T. (1986) Stroke Assessment: It's Time We All Spoke the Same Language. *Geriatric Medicine*, May, 11–12.

Wade, D. T. (1987) Who Looks after Stroke Patients? *British Journal of Hospital Medicine*, March, 201–4.

Wade, D. T. (1989) Organization of Stroke Care Services. *Clinical Rehabilitation*, **3**, 227–33.

Wade, D. T. (1992) Acute Stroke: Treatment and Rehabilitation,. *Hospital Update*, May, 370–75.

Wade, D. T. and Langton Hewer, R. (1987) Epidemiology of Some Neurological Diseases. *International Rehabilitation Medicine*, **8**, (3), 129–37.

Wade, D. T., Skilbeck, C. E., Langton Hewer, R. and Wood, V. A. (1984) Therapy After Stroke: Amounts, Determinants and Effects, *International Rehabilitation Medicine*, **6**, 105–10.

Wade, D.T., Wood, V. A. and Langton Hewer, R. (1985) Use of Hospital Resources by Acute Stroke Patients *Journal of the Royal College of Physicians of London*, **19**, (1), 48–52.

Walton, G. (1990) Physiotherapy. In Hewlett, J. (ed.) *Keyguide to Information Sources in Paramedical Sciences*, pp. 73–87, London and New York, Mansell.

Weddell, R., Oddy, M. and Jenkins, D. (1980) Social Adjustment after Rehabilitation: a Two-Year Follow-Up of Patients with Severe Head Injury. *Psychological Medicine*, **10**, 257–63.

Weiner, B. B. (1968) Curriculum Development for Children with Brain Damage. In Bortner, M. (ed.) *Evaluation and Education of Children with Brain Damage*, Illinois, Charles C. Thomas.

White, R. (1978) *Social Change and the Development of the Nursing Profession*, London, Henry Kimpton.

Whitehead, A. N. (1922) *The Aims of Education*, London, Benn.

Whiting, S., Lincoln, N. B., Bhavani, G. and Cockburn, T. (1985) *Rivermead Perceptual Assessment Battery*, NFER-Nelson, Windsor.

Wilson, B., Cockburn, J. and Baddeley, A. (1985) *Rivermead Behavioural Memory Test*, Reading, Thames Valley Test Company.

Wilson, W. and Laidler, P (1990) How Teams can Achieve 'Skill-Blend'. *Speech Therapy in Practice*, December, pp. 7–8.

Winterton, L. and Haldane, L. (1988) Methods of Record Keeping. In Squires, A. (ed.) *Rehabilitation of the Older Patient*, 249–63.

Wirz, S., Skinner, C. and Dean, E. (1992) *Revised Edinburgh Functional Communication Profile*, Oxon, UK, Winslow.

Yura, H. and Walsh, M. B. (1967) *The Nursing Process*, Norwalk, Appleton-Century-Crofts.

Index